Dedication

This book is dedicated to the patients we have served. They have taught us about courage and trust and have allowed us to function as their advocates. We have been reminded repeatedly of the importance of honesty in tandem with compassion and we are better practitioners for it.

CHAPTER 11 / Pain in Infants and Children

Valerie S. Hammel, RN, MSN
Pediatric Clinical Nurse Specialist
Kaiser Permanente
Fontana, CA

Cheryl Cahill, RN, MSN
Epilepsy Nurse Coordinator
Children's Hospital
Boston, MA

Cynthia Levin, RN, MA
Clinical Specialist, Psychiatric Nursing of Children
    and Adolescents
Children's Hospital
Boston, MA

CHAPTER 12 / Pain in Older Adults

Roger A. Weise, MD
Consultant in Geriatric Medicine
Alexian Brothers Medical Center
Elk Grove, IL

Rita Epsom, RN, MS
Geriatric Clinical Nurse Specialist
Alexian Brothers Medical Center
Elk Grove, IL

CHAPTER 13 / Substance Abuse: Assessment and Treatment
Challenges

Mary L. Cunningham, RN, MSN
Clinical Nurse Specialist, Pain and Symptom Management
M. D. Anderson Cancer Center
Houston, TX

Preface

Pain is a common experience for most people. Even with the emphasis by professional organizations, government agencies, regulatory and accrediting bodies and consumer groups, effective pain management continues to be elusive. While some pain experiences are brief and easily endured, there are many that are so severe and/or so constant that they penetrate the very fiber of people's lives. One would think that with major technological advances and new drug discoveries, cutting-edge pain management would be available to relieve this suffering. Effective pain management interventions are, indeed, available but not consistently applied. The gap between "what could be" and "what is" exists because of basic lack of knowledge and well-established biases on the part of many healthcare professionals. It is the intent of this publication to rally healthcare professionals to this challenge and support them by providing a resource that is easily accessed in individual clinical situations. It is hoped that by changing individual beliefs and practices, the collective picture of pain management will be positively affected. As professionals, we must hold each other accountable and collaborate in such a way that effective pain management becomes the norm. Compassionate patient care demands no less.

The authors of this publication have long been committed to improving the management of pain through educating practitioners and influencing policy. Each has a track record of providing clinically relevant information and tools for the clinicians at the bedside and in the field. Ruth Kingdon received her BSN from Northwestern University, Chicago and MSN from Loyola University, Chicago. Prepared as a clinical nurse specialist, Ruth has served as faculty of nursing programs at both Ravenswood Hospital and William Rainey Harper College in Illinois and directed nursing education at Alexian Brothers Medical Center there. She has co-authored several professional publications on both management and clinical topics (including a drug handbook for nurses), which are evidence of her personal belief that management and education are interwoven—development of people being the commitment that precedes achievement of quality. In her administrative role, Ruth has been able to encourage pain management education, support professionals and approve local programs to advance the cause of effective pain management in underserved populations.

Karen Stanley obtained her BSN from the University of Alabama, Birmingham and her MSN from the University of California, San Francisco. Karen has a dual background in oncology nursing and pain management. In addition to her position as a clinical nurse specialist in pain and symptom management, Karen is Assistant Clinical Professor in the School of Nursing Graduate Program at University of California, Los Angeles. She is certified as an advanced oncology nurse, is an active leader in the Oncology Nursing Society, and is a key individual in the management of pain for Kaiser Fontana's Hospice and Home Health patients. In addition to her exemplary work with complex pain challenges Karen spends much of her time sharing her expertise with other healthcare professionals, not only at the medical center but throughout the United States and other countries. She has participated in Pain Management Delegations to Russia, Hungary, Czechoslovakia, Singapore, Vietnam, and Thailand. Karen has been nationally recognized for her advocacy of patients in end of life situations, having appeared on PBS with a renowned panel on this topic and presently participating in the development of a national white paper on this critical issue.

Robert Kizior received his B.S. in Pharmacy from the College of Pharmacy at the University of Illinois, Chicago. Formerly adjunct faculty at William Rainey Harper College, Robert has provided several pharmacology courses to nurses. In addition to his position as Education Coordinator for the Department of Pharmacy, Robert has reviewed, consulted on or published various pharmacology publications, including a drug handbook for nurses. He has had responsibility for diverse areas of patient care, including Intensive Care, Skilled Nursing, Medical/Surgical Nursing, Oncology, Pediatrics and support to the OR Pharmacy satellite.

In keeping with the intent of the authors to help clinicians in day-to-day practice, this publication has followed a user-friendly format, with a conversational writing style throughout. There is a logical order of material, with chapters progressing from simple, fundamental concepts to specific applications in defined populations. In all chapters, content is field focused, i.e., presented in a way that is applicable to real life situations. This handbook provides basic principles of chronic and acute pain management in diverse populations. Relief of pain in specific populations includes infants and children, older adults, and those with a history of substance abuse. The latter is of particular interest since this population is growing and has had relatively little attention in the general healthcare setting. Individual chapters address the needs of patients with acute, chronic nonmalignant, and cancer pain. A newer population whose relief of pain has had little special emphasis are those with HIV/ AIDS; this topic is covered within the cancer pain chapter.

The physiology chapter is absolutely unique. Unlike traditional, dry reviews of physiology, this chapter has a fresh approach, combining drug actions to the physiology at each step. This results in a very clear understanding for the reader of how drugs may best be used in various clinical situations. A special feature is the use of a "Clinical Accountabilities" section at the end of all appropriate chapters which captures the major clinical accountabilities discussed in the chapter and lists them for both summary and emphasis. A striking advantage is the number and usability of tables for quick reference. An equianalgesic conversion table provides excellent guidelines in modifying drugs for better patient response. The substance abuse chapter includes an extensive table of the most commonly abused drugs, signs and symptoms, withdrawal, etc. In addition, there are many smaller but quite useful tables and figures throughout. Within the pediatric chapter are plans of care for both acute and chronic pain management. These have been developed by staff and are in actual use at the present time. Several case studies have been included to help the reader transfer the theory into common clinical encounters. Walking through these tangible situations may help understanding and retention. It is hoped that this clinical reference will become worn with use and that patients will benefit from the new learnings.

Ruth T. Kingdon
Karen J. Stanley
Robert J. Kizior

Acknowledgments

Our thanks to David C. Ianacone, MD and Betty R. Ferrell, PhD, FAAN for sharing their clinical expertise.

Contents

Notice

Pain Management is an ever-changing field. Standard safety precautions must be followed, but as new research and clinical experience broaden our knowledge, changes in treatment and drug therapy become necessary or appropriate. Readers are advised to check the product information currently provided by the manufacturer of each drug to be administered to verify the recommended dose, the method and duration of administration, and contraindications. It is the responsibility of the treating physician relying on experience and knowledge of the patient. Neither the Publisher nor the editor assumes any responsibility for any injury and/or damage to persons or property.

The Publisher

1
Introduction

Quality care, patient rights, caring, ethical decisions—these are not new words in health care; they have been woven into the fabric of patient care, as any professional can attest. What is new is the attempt to define them within the context of the technological, informational age in which we live. What do these words really mean to the patient and to the clinicians? How is their essence perpetuated in everyday practice in hospitals, in patient homes, in clinics or offices, in skilled nursing facilities? Laying aside extraordinary challenges, the overwhelming majority of care situations are evaluated on how well they meet the basic needs of patients. One measure of how well these elemental needs are being met is the efficacy of pain management. Effective pain management reflects caring, is a core component of quality care, and is a fundamental patient right.

So, how would pain management score on this quality grid? Without that moment of truth, one might smile, remembering the crude efforts to alleviate suffering of years past. Viewing those efforts from the informational age, one might tend to discredit their efficacy and feel a certain superiority of modern-day advancements. Yet, strangely enough, despite all the achievements of health care, effective pain management is still an elusive goal. The scorecard for pain management would not be one to celebrate; on the contrary, it should be a wake-up call for every health care practitioner in the country.

In a time of organ transplants, genetic research, laparoscopic surgery, and highly computerized noninvasive testing, why do patients still experience unrelieved pain? It seems incomprehensible that pain, the common denominator of so many illnesses and disorders (or the procedures to correct them), has received relatively little attention. It is equally puzzling that health care professionals who are sensitive to patients'

1

needs have not risen en masse to challenge the status quo. Nor has the link between inadequate pain control, health status, and costs become a national issue despite the interest in health care reform at the highest levels in the country. What is missing? Or rather, why is it being missed?

Major breakthroughs occurred in health care, but pain management went relatively unnoticed until approximately the mid-1970s. Then, despite research that introduced better ways of handling pain situations, the passion of a number of pioneers in several fields, the proliferation of new analgesics, and the introduction of successful techniques such as patient-controlled analgesia (PCA) and epidural analgesia, preventable pain experiences continued. Although there is still much to be learned about pain, it is clear that the present void is at the grassroots level. It is a deficit in the knowledge and application of what *is* known—by the clinicians caring for people everywhere and, more important, a deficit in understanding that significance. This is not intended as a fingerpointing exercise, but rather a cry to arousal, a plea for commitment to finding a better way.

Clinicians must understand and move beyond their own barriers that obstruct appropriate pain treatment. It is true that physicians and nurses have not been adequately prepared in their educational courses to understand pain fully and manage it successfully. In addition, they and other professionals have been influenced by their own cultural and personal beliefs about pain and conditioned over time by common myths. Like patients, caregivers harbor beliefs about pain that form impediments to proper management. Some cultures hold in high esteem the uncomplaining endurance of pain, a fact that prevents effective communication about the experience and adequate intervention. There may be a religious or cultural belief or a judgment call that interprets pain as punishment to be accepted as atonement for a past offense, real or imagined. Perhaps a person's role in society causes one to be "macho" or a "good patient" who does not complain, and beliefs of clinicians mirror those of the patients, or at least accept them unquestioningly. Clinicians develop their own professional biases about when a patient should or should not experience pain or how much pain is "reasonable." Most profoundly in the realm of the clinician is the bias that patients must exhibit certain behaviors to have their pain recognized and treated.

The myths about medications have particular impact on the thinking of clinicians. Fearing that increasing analgesics to attain pain relief will cause addiction or that opioids for extreme pain must be artificially limited to prevent overdose and possible death, many clinicians deny patients rightful and appropriate pain management. Chronic pain is particularly susceptible to biases. Few clinicians understand the multidimensional nature of chronic pain and the ramifications on patients' lives. Misconceptions about chronic pain, as well as tolerance versus addiction, can lead to withholding medications from patients who appear to be manipulating the health care team to gain more medications. In addition, clinicians who selected health care to relieve suffering and save lives may not be able to face their own inadequacy in managing intractable pain. They become frustrated, perceiving their care to be a failure, a perception that often results in avoiding the patient and exacerbates pain mismanagement.

Although education must be revised to address the pain management issue for the future, it cannot remain an excuse for practicing clinicians. One of the characteristics of a true professional is commitment to ongoing education and continuing improvement. It is therefore in full keeping with professional obligation to suggest that clinicians everywhere take ownership of their own knowledge about pain management and adapt their practices accordingly.

Once there is a commitment, then what? The first step is to examine one's own beliefs and biases, recognizing them as just that—one individual's personal perspective. It is difficult to change one's beliefs, but professionals have learned to use knowledge and research as a basis for establishing new thinking and determining standards by which care is given. Too often, as new learning occurs, old learnings are forgotten. It is imperative that the sophistication of high technology does not negate the value of high-touch, basic nursing *care*. The art of comfort is as important as the advancements of science. Action is the next step: taking the initiative to read the literature, to learn about research, to question, to identify resources for special needs. The third step is to maintain courage of conviction. The latter may be the most difficult part because once educated and aligned with state-of-the-art pain management, one may find that other professionals have not moved forward—or out of the road. To accept less than optimal pain relief is to accept less than optimal patient care. So, one must not only learn, but also share learnings with colleagues and partners and advocate on behalf of patients.

As health care professionals admit their own biases, they will also expose the biases and confusion of society as a whole. In a society that has struggled with the abuse of marijuana for three decades, therapeutic use is still withheld in legitimate situations. In fear and ignorance of drug abuse, patients have been labeled "addicts" when they became tolerant of analgesics taken for legitimate pain relief. Those struggling with intractable pain have been left, as the lepers were in Molokai, to suffer their days quietly in order to avoid "overmedicating" or "developing addiction" or simply because the answers were not known. But, today those myths have no place. Tolerance has been distinguished from addiction, chronic pain has been effectively treated with opioids; overmedicating has been separated from the need of those in unrelieved pain. This is a new and enlightened day.

In addition to the education and championship of clinicians, patient participation is needed. For too long, this country has depended passively on the healthcare system and the professionals within it to work miracles, create cures. Now, finally, people are beginning to accept responsibility for their own health. It is both refreshing and exciting to see patients begin to question their treatment, make decisions, and participate in their own health. But healthcare professionals ought not to accept this change passively—they should embrace this monumental shift of control, which will truly determine the health of the nation. This is a major turning point in the pain battle, because clinicians need the involvement of patients to achieve optimal pain management. One of the key points of this publication is that patients must take control of their pain and the quality of their existence. They cannot do that alone, but with the help of knowledgeable clinicians, they can change their pain responses and ultimately the quality of the lives they live. The cumulative results of such individual pain victories affect the quality and cost of care on a global level.

Fortunately, several agencies and organizations have made a commitment to and are moving forward on behalf of optimal pain management. One of eight agencies of the U.S. Public Health Service, the Agency for Health Care Policy and Research (AHCPR) has developed and disseminated clinical practice guidelines for acute and cancer pain management. In so doing, AHCPR is contributing to the establishment of national standards for pain relief. Pain research and education have been advanced by the Oncology Nursing Society, the American Pain Society, and the National Cancer Institute, among others. The National Committee on Quality Assurance is developing "report cards" on the efficacy of patient care. The Joint Commission for the Accreditation of Healthcare Organizations (JCAHO) has included effective pain management within their standards for accreditation. Greater scrutiny of patient rights and care efficacy by governmental agencies, purchasers, and consumers will increase the focus on what constitutes quality care and, within that definition, effective pain management.

These efforts serve as a catalyst for improving pain experiences. However, they should not be the driving force in and of themselves. Healthcare institutions need to set the standards for effective pain management within their organizations. This can be achieved by developing pain clinics and/or pain management teams and through the expectation that all professionals collaborate on behalf of patients. Health care professionals have always prided themselves on setting high standards, demanding improved practice, and advancing the quality of care. In effect, clinicians and the professions they represent have demonstrated leadership in healthcare. Now is the time for that same professional commitment and energy to be directed toward the long-standing pain issue. With individual commitment and team collaboration, effective pain management is within grasp. Pain relief needs to be a priority for each healthcare profession and owned by every clinician to effect real change.

Time is pressing. Issues in care continue to surface, challenging the moral fiber of our society and of health care professionals. The rising costs of health care have generated concern for the viability of the health care system and created anxiety throughout the nation regarding access to care. Clifton Gaus, administrator of AHCPR, stated in a 1995 interview that "better quality often costs less," as demonstrated by hospitals decreasing costs through effective pain management. Research has shown that effective pain management results in shorter recovery time and better outcomes. Mismanagement of chronic pain causes overuse of all areas of the health care systems. According to the American Pain Society, 50 million people are disabled by pain in this country, many of whom suffer from chronic pain. Consider the psychological devastation and the impact on the lives of those individuals and their families. Here are opportunities to reduce costs while significantly improving quality of life.

Moral and ethical questions abound and will continue to come up. Some are complex and difficult to resolve, but others simply lay open ineffectual treatment. The controversial issue of assisted suicide has exposed a void in care that health care professionals must recognize and act upon. That void is the inadequate relief of pain and suffering in the terminally ill, the anguish of which makes death a more acceptable choice. For professionals dedicated to life and the comfort of those who cannot be saved, there is only one answer—more knowledgeable, aggressive, and compassionate treatment of suffering.

The challenges are great, but the possibilities exciting and rewarding. The purpose of this handbook is to demystify pain management, for when all is said and done, it is the clinician at the bedside or in the field who will make the difference.

2

The Physiology and Experience of Pain

An unpleasant sensory and emotional experience associated with actual and potential tissue damage, and described in terms of such damage—International Association for the Study of Pain, Subcommittee of Taxonomy

and/or

Pain is whatever the experiencing person says it is and exists whenever he says it does—McCaffery

Pain is a complex, biopsychosocial phenomenon that occurs among widely diverse groups of patient populations. It is a primary sensation that serves to protect the human organism against further damage from external and internal occurrences. The current literature provides a relatively comprehensive understanding of the physiologic mechanisms and pathways of pain, but the individual's perception of pain and of its meaning develops over time and with experience. The International Association for the Study of Pain (1979) acknowledges in its definition the sensory and emotional facets of the pain experience. McCaffery's (1979) definition reminds us that pain is a highly individualized experience whose assessment centers on the patient's self-report. Historical experience has taught us that pain can exist with no identifiable pathophysiologic etiology. We also have learned that individuals with similar physiologic circumstances do not necessarily have similar pain experiences.

The conceptual incorporation of patient self-report into the working definition of pain acknowledges both the subjective nature of the pain experience and the collaborative relationship between the patient and health care provider. However, these definitions do not take into account those human beings who are incapable of self-report, such as newborns and infants, small children, mentally retarded, comatose, or demented patients, or verbally handicapped individuals. Although the sensation of pain and subsequent verbal report are related and sequential events, those who cannot communicate effectively are essentially excluded. It has been suggested that the current definitions of pain deserve further attention. It is certainly true that nonverbal behavioral information is used when assessing pain in the aforementioned patient populations, but many clinicians believe that the incorporation of biologic and behavioral reactions would define the pain experience more appropriately.

PHYSIOLOGY

There are numerous ways to approach the pain experience, but an understanding of the basic anatomic structures and the physiologic processes that transmit the pain signal provides a framework for appropriate assessment and intervention. The structures and processes that are activated when an injury occurs together transmit the pain signal from the damaged site to the brain. An ascending system of nerve fibers carries that signal from the peripheral to the central nervous system where the pain experience is recognized. Physiologic processes, including the activity of neurotransmitters, are operative at multiple sites along this structural pathway to aid in conveying the signal. This process is referred to as **nociception.**

Nociceptive Process

The nociceptive process begins at the peripheral level. When damage occurs, biochemical agents that initiate or sensitize the nociceptive response are released. These agents include potassium, substance P, bradykinin, and prostaglandin, among others. Potassium is released from damaged cells, substance P from unmyelinated nociceptors, and bradykinin from plasma

Modulation
↓
Injury → Transduction → Transmission → Perception

FIGURE 2–1   *The Nociceptive Process*

leaking from surrounding blood vessels. Prostaglandin has many functions, one of which is to sensitize nerve endings at the peripheral level. When trauma occurs, enzymes convert phospholipids, a cellular membrane component, to arachidonic acid and subsequently to prostaglandin. The initial injury provokes a series of physiologic events (Figure 2–1).

Transduction

The initial stimulus (injury) provokes primary afferent fibers involved in pain (nociceptors). This stimulus triggers an action potential in those fibers character- ized by depolarization (exchange of sodium and potas- sium ions across the neuronal membrane). In essence the fiber is "charged." It is at this point that pharma- cologic agents known as membrane stabilizers (anti- convulsants, such as Tegretol®, Dilantin®, and anes- thetics, such as Marcaine®) can be effective. They interfere with the depolarization process by blocking the ion channels and subsequently stopping the resultant action potential. Anticonvulsants seem to be particularly effective in suppressing the sharp, shoot- ing pain sensation as their effects on the membrane reduce the ability of axons to act quickly.

Transmission

The action potential (pain signal) ascends along the neuronal path from the source of the pain to the cerebral cortex in several steps, much like a relay race:

1. The primary afferent neuron carries the signal from the injured site to the dorsal horn of the spinal cord.

2. The primary afferent neuron synapses with the spinothalamic tract neurons in the dorsal horn;

the message is relayed across this synapse via neurotransmitters, such as substance P.

3. The spinothalamic tract neurons continue to transmit the pain signal upward through the spinal cord, which contains large quantities of opioid receptors.

4. Spinothalamic tract neurons ascend to the thalamus in the midbrain and from there to various areas of the brain.

Perception

Perception is the actual pain experience that occurs when the action potential reaches the areas of the brain that allow recognition of the pain sensation (somatosensory cortex, association cortex, frontal lobe, and the limbic system). In addition to relaying the pain signal from the injured site to the brain, the body also has a marked ability to inhibit the transmission of that signal while it is in process, a little like erecting a wall across a road to stop traffic. This process is referred to as *modulation.* It occurs in a separate central nervous system structure from the ascending pathway that carries the signal to the brain.

Modulation

Modulation is a restraining of the nociceptive process. A *descending* system of nerve fibers originating in the pons and medulla releases biochemicals (e.g., serotonin, norepinephrine, and noradrenergic substances) within the dorsal horn and hinders the ascending pain signal before it is recognized in the higher brain centers.

The release of serotonin, norepinephrine, and noradrenergic substances has analgesic pharmacologic implications. The body, under normal conditions, will release serotonin from neuronal terminals. The serotonin subsequently binds to a nearby neuron, is released, and then absorbed back into the original neuron. Tricyclic antidepressants (e.g., Elavil®, Norpramin®, Tofranil®, Pamelor®) have demonstrated analgesic effects that are independent of their antidepressant activity. They prevent the reuptake of serotonin, causing more to be available in the synaptic area and thus inhibit the further relay of the ascending pain signal. This process imitates the body's endogenous modulatory activity. Tricyclic antidepressants seem to be most helpful for pain of postherpetic neuralgia or diabetic neuralgia, conditions characterized by dull aching or burning.

Another set of neurons within the midbrain, the noradrenergic neurons, also descend to the spinal cord and inhibit relay of the pain signal at the dorsal horn level. There are significant quantities of α_2-noradrenergic receptors in the spinal cord. The noradrenergic neurons secrete substances that bind to those receptors and inhibit the relay of the ascending pain signal. Clonidine, a noradrenergic agonist, imitates this activity and modulates the ascending pain message. Significant clinical work has been done in the area of intraspinal clonidine. See Chapter 5 for further details.

As the nociceptive process is reviewed, it is clear that the message is relayed through a series of ascending nerve fibers. The action potential (pain signal) must not only travel through those fibers, but must also cross the neuronal synapse. Substances known as neurotransmitters serve as the biochemical bridge between one neuron and the next. Because neurotransmitters assist in the relay of the pain signal, pharmacologic management of pain may involve the inhibition of those neurotransmitters. When the action potential in the primary afferent neuron reaches the dorsal horn of the spinal cord, receptors on the end of the neuron relay the pain message to the secondary neuron in the spinothalamic tract by releasing substance P. The substance P crosses the synapse and binds to receptors on the secondary neuron. The pain message is relayed along the neuronal path through the central nervous system in this manner. The dorsal horn also contains significant quantities of opioid receptors. When the patient receives an opioid analgesic, such as morphine, those opioids will attach to the receptors and inhibit the release of substance P, thus inhibiting the transmission of the pain signal. The large quantity of opioid receptors in the spinal cord provides the rationale for intraspinal administration of opioids. See Chapter 5 for more information.

Types of Pain

Given that the pain signal is transmitted and modulated by the peripheral and central nervous systems, damage to those systems can alter the nature of the pain experience. **Nociceptive pain** is defined as the process wherein the pain signal is transmitted by a *normal/intact* nervous system. It can be somatic (arising from general body structures, especially musculoskeletal) or visceral (arising from autonomic fibers in the smooth muscle of the internal organs). It is characterized as heavy, dull, sharp, aching, and/or throbbing in nature. Examples include headache, postoperative incisional pain, muscle spasms, broken bones, and some kinds of cancer pain.

Neuropathic pain differs from nociceptive pain in that the pain signal is transmitted by a *damaged* nervous system. The damage, including cutting, crushing, and/or compression injuries to the nervous system, as well as exposure to neurotoxic drugs or viral agents, causes both structural and chemical changes. Changes may occur at multiple sites in the nervous system, including the area of damage, the spinal cord, or the brain. Those changes trigger abnormalities in the way the pain signal is transmitted to the brain and thus alter the nature of the pain experience. Potential mechanisms of neuropathic pain include spontaneous discharge in the regenerating nerve, spontaneous activity in the dorsal root ganglion, and/or a degeneration in the modulatory systems.

Neuropathic pain is typically described as burning, shooting, or electrical in nature, although it is so different from other pain experiences that patients may have difficulty in describing the sensations. Examples include postherpetic neuralgia, brachial plexopathy, diabetic neuropathy, phantom limb pain, and trigeminal neuralgia.

A single pathophysiologic condition may have nociceptive and neuropathic components, such as cancer of the lung with invasion of the brachial plexus.

These nociceptive and neuropathic factors determine the anatomic distribution and characteristics of the pain sensation, effective treatment interventions, and the chronicity of the pain experience. Historically, opioid analgesics have been perceived as effective when treating nociceptive pain and generally ineffective when treating neuropathic pain. Although patient responses to pharmacologic interventions do not always fit so neatly into this categorization (i.e., pain considered to be neuropathic in origin may respond to opioid analgesics), in reality neuropathic pain often does not respond to opioid intervention. As a result, other pharmacologic avenues have been explored to relieve neuropathic pain. Table 2–1 correlates pharmacologic interventions to pain physiology based on the mechanism of action of the drug. See Chapter 4 for a discussion of analgesic medications.

Opioid Receptor Sites

There are multiple endogenous (internally secreted) opioidlike substances and opioid receptor sites distributed throughout the central nervous system at the spinal and supraspinal levels and in the periphery. The three groups of endogenous opioid peptides, enkephalins, dynorphins, and β-endorphin, are released when the brain gives a signal. They attach to the opioid receptor site, that portion of the nerve cell to which the drug can bind, and block the transmission of the pain signal. There are three primary receptors: mu, kappa, and delta (refer to Table 2-2). Endorphin research suggests that multiple factors may increase or decrease their levels. Prolonged pain, recurrent stress, and prolonged use of opioids or alcohol will decrease their circulating levels. Brief pain or stress, physical exercise, massive trauma, some types of acupuncture, some types of transcutaneous electrical nerve stimulation (TENS) units, and sexual activity all can increase the circulating levels.

The opioid analgesic drugs mimic the actions of these naturally occurring peptides and attach to the

TABLE 2-1 *Clinical Implications of Pain Physiology*

PHARMACOLOGIC INTERVENTION	RATIONALE
NSAIDs	Traumatized cells release prostaglandins that sensitize primary afferent fibers; NSAIDs inhibit prostaglandin synthesis, thereby blocking pain in the periphery
Opioids (systemic and intraspinal)	Bind to receptors in the dorsal horn and inhibit release of neurotransmitters (e.g., substance P), subsequently interfering with transmission of pain message
Membrane stabilizers Anesthetics Anticonvulsants	Block ion channels, preventing action potential generation (pain signal) along neuronal path; very useful for neuropathic pain
Antidepressants	Inhibit reuptake of serotonin into neuronal fibers, thus making more serotonin available in the synaptic area and inhibiting nociceptive transmission (pain message). A modulatory response. May be useful for neuropathic pain
Noradrenergic agonists	Attach to α_2-noradrenergic receptors in the dorsal horn of the spinal cord and inhibit nociceptive transmission. A modulatory response

receptor sites in the same manner with varying levels of affinity and for varied periods of time. By attaching to those receptors, they inhibit the release of substance P, a powerful neurotransmitter, and thus interfere with the transmission of the pain signal. The opioid's affinity for the receptor site and the time it remains bound at that site affect both the degree and duration of analgesic relief.

Opioid agonist drugs stimulate activity when they attach to a receptor site, whereas opioid antagonist drugs block activity at the receptor site. Thus, morphine, an agonist drug that binds at the μ-receptor site, will provide pain relief, but naloxone, an antagonist drug that also binds at the μ-receptor site, will block pain relief by interfering with the agonist drug that is attached to those same receptor sites. In essence, it displaces the agonist drug from the receptor. Mixed agonist-antagonist drugs (e.g., pentazocine [Talwin®], butorphanol [Stadol®], nalbuphine [Nubain®]) affect more than one type of opioid receptor. They demonstrate agonist activity and antagonist activity at one or more receptors.

The side effect profiles of the varied opioid analgesics are well known. The same opioid receptors that modulate analgesia also can trigger respiratory depression, constipation, euphoria, sedation, physical dependence, and tolerance (Table 2–2). See Chapter 4 for more details.

Tolerance, Physical Dependence, and Psychological Dependence (Addiction)

Misunderstanding about tolerance of, and physical and psychological dependence (addiction) on opioid analgesics interferes with adequate pain management by health care professionals and consumers. There is no doubt that major societal problems have occurred as a result of psychological dependence (addiction), but the fear that *appropriate* use of opioids causes psychological dependence is not based on any scientific evidence. Tolerance and physical dependence are separate, involuntary physiologic occurrences. Psychological dependence, although commonly believed to be

TABLE 2-2   *Opioid Receptor Site Activity*

Opioid Receptor Site	Activity	Agonist Activity	Antagonist Activity
Mu	Spinal/supraspinal analgesia Respiratory depression Physical dependence Tolerance Decreased GI motility Euphoria Sedation	Morphine Methadone (Dolophine®) Fentanyl (Sublimaze®, Duragesic®) Hydromorphone (Dilaudid®) Meperidine (Demerol®) Codeine	Naloxone (Narcan®) Naltrexone (Trexan®) Partial: butorphanol (Stadol®) Nalbuphine (Nubain®) Pentazocine (Talwin®)
Kappa	Spinal level analgesia Sedation Little respiratory depression Little physical dependence	Butorphanol (Stadol®) Buprenorphine (Buprenex®) Nalbuphine (Nubain®) Pentazocine (Talwin®)	Naloxone (Narcan®) Naltrexone (Trexan®)
Delta	Analgesia Less respiratory depression No physical dependence	Deltorphins*	Naloxone-type drugs

*Highly selective delta agonists do not penetrate the blood–brain barrier and therefore must be administered intrathecally or intracerebroventricularly.

16

demonstrated by tolerance and/or physical dependence, is neither and should be examined separately.

Tolerance

Tolerance is an involuntary, physiologic behavior that occurs after repeated exposure to an opioid analgesic. It is evidenced by decreased pain relief at a stable or escalating opioid analgesic dose. Tolerance

- Does not occur with short-term exposure to opioid analgesics.
- Is more likely to occur with chronic use for malignant pain.
- Is first evidenced by decreased duration of relief, then decreased degree of relief.
- *Does not mean that the patient is psychologically dependent (addicted).*

Physical Dependence

Physical dependence is an involuntary, physiologic behavior that is evidenced by the occurrence of withdrawal symptoms if the opioid is abruptly stopped or an opioid antagonist is administered. Physical dependence

- Occurs only after repeated opioid administration.
- Produces in most instances withdrawal symptoms so mild that they are not recognized and require no treatment. Significant exposure to substantial opioid dosages may result in the need to taper the drug rather than discontinue it abruptly.
- *Does not mean that the patient is psychologically dependent (addicted).*

Psychological Dependence

Psychological dependence is a chronic disorder evidenced by overwhelming involvement with obtaining and using a drug for its psychic effects, not for approved medical reasons. It results in physical, psychological, and/or social harm to the user. Psychological dependence is characterized by

- Active, compulsive drug seeking
- Tendency to relapse even after physical withdrawal subsides
- The fact that duration of opioid therapy does not increase its incidence

Although withdrawal symptoms are similar in the physically dependent and the psychologically dependent (addicted) individual, the latter is distinguished by the loss of personal control over drug use.

There is significant controversy in the current pain management arena about the use of opioid analgesics in the chronic nonmalignant pain patient population. Part of the controversy centers on the dependence liability of opioid analgesics. Concerned clinicians focus on the likelihood that the euphoria commonly seen in the substance abuse population will "lure" patients into psychological dependence, even though there may be no other predisposing factors. Contradictory evidence to this supposition is seen in postoperative pain, cancer pain, and normal volunteer patient populations who do not experience euphoria subsequent to the administration of opioid analgesics. In addition, other situational and social factors implicated in the predisposition to substance abuse are unusual in the typical medical patient. Although there are numerous surveys of patients without prior opioid use who were administered opioids for pain relief and demonstrated no addictive behavior, consensus is lacking on this treatment approach. The task at hand remains to identify those patient populations that would most likely benefit from this approach without complications.

THE PAIN EXPERIENCE

The two definitions of pain articulated at the beginning of this chapter are generic enough to be inclusive of both the acute and chronic pain experiences. The acute versus chronic categorization is differentiated by the expected trajectory of the pain experience. Chapters 8 and 9 will provide more detail on the nature of acute and chronic pain. As the pain experience is examined, it is important to remember that the short-term, self-limited nature and progressive resolution of the acute pain experience has more limited implications than the long-term, often difficult-to-treat, possibly intractable nature of the chronic pain experience. Chronic pain can quickly deplete an individual's physical and emotional resources. It can immobilize the individual, lead to physical disability and subsequent loss of employment, significantly impact daily activities, interrupt sleeping habits, and interfere with interpersonal relationships. As the nature of the pain experience becomes more complex, the impact on the individual becomes more extensive.

Melzack and Casey (1968) have suggested three major dimensions to the pain experience: sensory-discriminative, motivational-affective, and cognitive-evaluative. This framework recognizes *affective* or *emotional factors* as a central component of the pain experience. It has long been understood that anxiety, fear, apprehension, and depression, among others, can markedly affect the pain experience and be affected by it. For instance, anticipatory anxiety can heighten the pain experience and subsequent pain behavior. The filtering of the sensory component of the pain experience through an emotional grid colors the experience for each individual.

Cognitive and behavioral factors also affect the pain experience. Multiple experiments have demonstrated that when the individual's attention is focused on the pain sensation, its intensity can be exacerbated. Pain expression is a behavior that is molded by learning experiences. Personal rewards associated with pain behavior (e.g., more attention and/or sympathy) can increase the frequency and intensity of expression (operant learning or conditioning). The provision of structured learning sessions has demonstrated that educating patients about what they can expect during a pain-producing intervention can decrease the pain's intensity and control pain behaviors. Social learning or modeling allows the individual to learn by imitation.

Children are particularly receptive to this type of learning experience and will model their pain behaviors on the behavior they observe in family members and friends.

The *meaning* attributed to the pain and/or suffering also affects pain behavior. Foreboding circumstances associated with the underlying etiology of the pain can trigger a "why me" response as the individual attempts to identify the purpose of the experience. The pain experience can threaten beliefs about control and self-image. Many individuals fear becoming incapacitated and being viewed as such by family and friends. The perception that there is no personal control over the pain produces extreme anxiety and a sense of helplessness that may drive the individual to behave frantically and often inappropriately.

The individual pain experience is intricately linked to the *social environment* in which it occurs. Others' responses to pain and pain behavior, whether communicated verbally or behaviorally, affect future behavior. Social isolation can exacerbate pain behaviors. *Culture*, a pattern of customs, beliefs, and values common to members of a specific group, also has an impact on the pain experience. The individual's attitude is determined by the meaning of the pain experience as defined by the culture, and the expression of pain is driven by cultural expectations.

Religious belief can have a significant impact on the meaning of the pain and the expected response to it. Historically, there has been great significance attached to pain and suffering. The pain may be associated with guilt-producing behavior and subsequent punishment or seen as atonement for past behaviors. For some, pain may be perceived as deserved retribution for prior actions.

The dimensions of the human *personality* or a predisposition to respond in certain ways can color how the individual adapts to or copes with the pain experience. As threat and stress are part of the pain experience, a response to the painful experience is generally consistent with the individual's response to any other stressful event.

Thus, the duration or intensity of pain a person is willing to endure is a unique response that is influenced by a multitude of physiologic and psychologic variables. Loeser (1982) proposed a model recognizing the variables that affect the pain experience and resultant behaviors. This model acknowledges that a *noxious stimulus* triggers the physiologic processes of pain signal transmission, which in turn cause **pain,** the perception and recognition of the sensation. The pain experience triggers and in return is affected by an emotional response to that sensation, which is articulated as **suffering.** The results of these interacting constructs are the visible **pain behaviors,** or what a person says or does that infers the experience of noxious stimulus.

The multidimensional nature of the pain experience and the essential role of motivational, affective, and environmental factors in driving pain behaviors provide the rationale for a comprehensive, multimodal, and multidisciplinary treatment approach. The complex nature of the chronic pain experience allows that the health care team cannot appropriately or successfully respond to pain from a physiologic standpoint alone. An effective, individualized approach should take into account the psychological and cultural attributes of the patient, as well as current pathophysiology.

BIBLIOGRAPHY

Anand, K.J.S., & Craig, K.D. (1996). New perspectives on the definition of pain. *Pain 67*(1), 3–6.

Basbaum, A.I. (1995). Insights into the development of opioid tolerance. *Pain 61*(3), 349–351.

Bonica, J.J. (1990). Anatomic and physiologic basis of nociception and pain. In J.J. Bonica (Ed.), *The management of pain* 2nd ed., (pp. 400–460). Philadelphia: Lea & Febiger.

Craig, K.D. (1993). The facial expression of pain: Better than a thousand words? *American Pain Society Journal 1,* 153–162.

Franz, D.N. (1993). Review of research on receptor pharmacology of pain and analgesia: Part one. *American Pain Society Bulletin* October/November, 10–13.

International Association for the Study of Pain, Subcommittee on Taxonomy. (1979). Part II. Pain terms: A current list with definitions and notes on usage. *Pain 6,* 249–252.

Loeser, J.D. (1982). Concepts of pain. In M. Stanton-Hicks & R. Boas (Eds.), *Chronic low back pain.* New York: Raven Press.

Maciewicz, R., Bouckoms, A., & Martin, J.B. (1985). Drug therapy of neuropathic pain. *The Clinical Journal of Pain 1,* 39–49.

McCaffery, M. (1979). *Nursing management of the patient with pain.* New York: J.B. Lippincott.

Melzack, R., & Casey, K.L. (1968). Sensory, motivational, and central control determinants of pain. In D.R. Kenshalo (Ed.), *The skin senses* (pp. 423–439). Springfield: Charles C. Thomas.

Morphine-A "local analgesic." (1995). In D.B. Carr (Ed.), *PAIN. Clinical updates, 3*(1), 1–4.

Paice, J.A. (1991). Unraveling the mystery of pain. *Oncology Nursing Forum, 18*(5), 843–849.

Pasternak, G.W. (1993). Pharmacological mechanisms of opioid analgesics. *Clinical Neuropharmacology 16*(1), 1–18.

Portenoy, R.K. (1990). Chronic opioid therapy in nonmalignant pain. *Journal of Pain and Symptom Management 5*(1 Suppl.), S46–S62.

Stein, C. (1991). Peripheral analgesic actions of opioids. *Journal of Pain and Symptom Management 6*(3), 119–124.

Zena, M., Strumpf, M., & Tryba, M. (1992). Long-term opioid therapy in patients with chronic nonmalignant pain. *Journal of Pain and Symptom Management 7*(2), 69–77.

3
Assessment

The assessment of pain, including characteristics, distinguishing features, and patterns, can be used for diagnostic purposes, defining treatment approaches, evaluating the efficacy of treatment, and identifying recurring or increasing pathology. A diagnostic assessment might include appropriate radiologic, neurologic, and nuclear medicine studies, serum assays, and a thorough history and physical examination. A detailed history is critical for an accurate assessment. Responses to queries soliciting the nature, location, onset, and pattern of the pain provide important diagnostic data. Patients should be allowed to use their own words. The diagnostician should avoid any hints of symptoms or diagnosis. This information may provide the clinician such a clear picture that diagnosis can be primarily determined from the symptoms alone. Many of the questions common to the initial diagnostic assessment should be repeated in the ongoing nursing assessment of that patient.

Treatment approaches are driven by the results of the diagnostic assessment. When existing pathology cannot be specifically identified, the pain may be treated based on its nature and location alone. Once treatment has begun, ongoing assessment of pain status as a measure of the treatment's efficacy can determine the direction of further intervention. Patients with pain secondary to a chronic illness that has been successfully treated or managed may experience a return to the pain state that indicates an increase in the current pathology, recurrent disease, or new pathology.

The nature of the pain experience determines the complexity of the assessment. Although pain can be a multifaceted and very complex biopsychosocial phenomenon, those patients with temporary, manageable pain secondary to a known etiology (e.g., surgery for a broken bone) may require only a limited assessment. That assessment would focus on the pre- and postanalgesic pain status to ensure the adequacy of analgesic relief. Conversely, the cancer patient with recurrent, widespread disease accompanied by significant pain requires a thorough assessment that includes both psychosocial and physiologic data. Pain that is chronic in nature, is intractable, and/or that comes from a life-threatening disease carries a far different meaning from an acute episode that will readily resolve when the tissue heals. The person as well as the pain must be assessed.

There are numerous reliable and valid multiple dimension self-report pain inventories available. The McGill Pain Questionnaire (Melzack, 1975) consists primarily of three major classes of word descriptors that measure sensory, affective, and evaluative domains. The long form (78-word descriptors) of this questionnaire takes about 20 minutes to complete, and the short form (15-word descriptors) requires between 2 and 5 minutes. They may be used for baseline and periodic evaluation but are not practical for frequent use. The Wisconsin Brief Pain Inventory (Daut, Cleeland, & Flanery, 1983) is a quick, multidimensional pain measure that has been used extensively in cancer and arthritis patient populations. It seems to be most appropriate for patients with progressive disease. The Memorial Pain Assessment Card (MPAC) rates pain, pain relief, and mood on visual analog scales and adds a set of descriptive words reflective of pain intensity (Fishman et al., 1986). It is short and easy to use, although patients may have trouble with the visual analog scale concept and with differentiating pain from pain relief.

A psychologic evaluation can be potentially useful in situations in which the pain interferes markedly with the patient's capacity to participate in routine activities, has adversely affected relationships with others, and/or in which the patient exhibits disproportionate emotional distress. It also may be appropriate when the patient uses the health care system excessively or continues to demand further tests or treatments after being informed they are not indicated. This evaluation is helpful in identifying the psychologic and behavioral factors involved in pain, suffering, and disability and may uncover pertinent historical psychosocial issues. It also may be useful in determining which psychologic and behavioral treatment strategies are indicated (Turner & Romano, 1990).

Components of the psychologic evaluation may include medical history and pain experience, patient identification of pain problem and treatment expectations, previous treatment and responses, drug and alcohol usage, behavioral analysis, vocational assessment and compensation/litigation status, social history, recent life stressors, and assessment of psychologic dysfunction.

The Minnesota Multiphasic Personality Inventory (MMPI; Hathaway & McKinley, 1967) is the most frequently used measure for assessing personality characteristics of chronic pain patients. Five hundred sixty-six true–false questions describe patients on three validity and ten clinical scales. Although it is used for its ability to predict response to therapeutic interventions for pain, it was developed for psychiatric populations, and thus its relevance to medical disorders is questioned. Inexperienced interpretation has resulted in chronic pain patients being told that they are depressed, anxious, overly concerned about their health, and exaggerating their problems (Helmes, 1994). The most important issues when considering use of the MMPI for patients with chronic pain are (1) whether the information gained is worth the effort expended; and (2) whether there are more efficient ways to obtain the same information. Helmes (1994) recommends the Personality Assessment Inventory (Morey, 1991) for its ability to distinguish the physiological symptoms of anxiety and depression from cognitive and emotional symptoms.

Nursing Assessment

The initial and ongoing nursing assessment is based on a simpler, less time-consuming structure. Two important basic premises should serve as a grid through which the data obtained from patient assessment is filtered.

Pain Is a Subjective Experience

Pain is what the experiencing person says it is, existing whenever the experiencing person says it does (McCaffery, 1979). The subjective nature of the pain experience demands adherence to the patient's evaluation as the initial standard. The patient, in fact, is the only one in the midst of that pain experience and thus is the expert. Health care providers may have different mindsets, expectations and/or life experiences. They may disagree with the patient's evaluation or may not believe in its truthfulness. The issue is complicated by the fact that pain cannot be seen and that identifiable pathophysiology may not always be present. Nevertheless, a professional code requires that the patient's statements be accepted and the patient treated respectfully and positively. The risk of being tricked or manipulated does not warrant disbelief or the withholding of analgesic interventions. When patients recognize that they are not believed, adversarial relationships can develop between the patient and health care team members.

As mentioned in Chapter 2, the assessment of pain in the patient who is unable to communicate effectively is a difficult issue. When the clinician cannot rely on the spoken word to document the presence of pain, behavioral characteristics become the patient's self-report. The clinician must be particularly alert to behavioral clues, such as restlessness in the comatose patient or crying in the neonate. See Chapters 11 and 12.

Acute versus Chronic Pain Assessment Requires Different Parameters

The nature and duration of the pain experience can trigger physiologic and psychologic adaptive mechanisms over time. Easily identifiable "common" pain behaviors may be absent as adaptation to the chronic pain experience occurs. The lack of pain expression does not mean that the pain is nonexistent. Physiologically, the autonomic nervous system adapts to the continued presence of pain, and expected parameters of increased blood pressure, pulse, and respirations, as well as diaphoresis may be absent. The individual also may adapt from a behavioral perspective. There may be a blank or normal facial expression, sleep or rest may be frequent, and attention may be focused on areas other than pain.

KEY POINT

As the patient with chronic pain adapts to the experience, observable signs diminish, although the pain's severity remains unchanged

---

The key point that observable signs may diminish while the intensity of pain remains the same bears repetition as most health care personnel use the acute model when evaluating the patient's pain status. To assess chronic pain using the acute model does both the patient and the health care provider an injustice. When patient veracity and acute versus chronic model differentiation become the standards, a more accurate and appropriate assessment can be conducted. A thorough initial nursing assessment should capture both the objective and subjective experiences.

DIMENSIONS

The dimensions of the pain experience provide both information on potential etiology and an overall "picture" of that experience. They include onset and duration; location; intensity and quality; relieving and exacerbating factors; and effects on activities of daily living. Identification of onset may provide etiologic clues. Duration establishes chronicity and can often provide insight into resultant behavior. The extent of the pain experience allows health care personnel to choose acute versus chronic assessment models.

It is important to remember that intensity is the most subjective of the dimensional characteristics. Intensity is measured by using a rating scale. These scales attempt to make a subjective experience as objective as possible. The consistent use of one rating approach provides a reliable source of comparison along the intervention continuum. Patients undergoing an analgesic trial period require ongoing and frequent assessment. Evaluation of pain intensity pre- and postanalgesic intervention can determine the efficacy of that intervention. To obtain accurate assessment data, it is important to use a scale that makes sense to the patient. Accuracy of assessment can be furthered by defining the parameters each time the scale is used until the patient is comfortable with that rating approach. As the clinician focuses on choosing the most appropriate scale, it is important to confirm that the patient understands the concept of pain. One can do this by having the patient describe a painful experience. When choosing the scale to be used, take into consideration the patient's level of comprehension, eyesight, and developmental status. It may be helpful to collaborate with the patient in choosing the most appropriate scale. See Chapter 11 on pediatric and Chapter 12 on aging populations about assessment modalities particular to those patients.

Scales that measure pain as self-report on a single dimension include visual analog scales, numerical rating scales, verbal descriptor scales, and the faces' scale. A *visual analog scale* (Figure 3–1) is comprised of a 10-centimeter line with endpoint descriptors. It is simple and quick and has been determined to be reliable and valid. However, the abstract nature of the concept makes it difficult for some, and it does require a new ruler for each use. For those who are unable to use a numerical scale, a visual analog scale may be helpful. Examples of these scales are included in the text. They are to serve only as examples and are not to be replicated for patient use as the dimensions may not

| No pain at all | _____ | Worst pain imaginable |

FIGURE 3–1   *Visual Analog Scale*
Instructions: Mark on the line above how strong your pain is right now.

| No pain at all | 0 | 1 | 2 | 3 | 4 | 5 | 6 | 7 | 8 | 9 | 10 | Worst pain imaginable |

FIGURE 3–2 *Numerical Rating Scale*
Instructions: Choose a number from 0 to 10 that indicates how strong your pain is right now.

be absolutely correct and thus compromise both the reliability and validity (Figure 3–1).

Numerical rating scales are quick, simple, and easy to use. The patient can point to, mark, or verbalize the number that corresponds to the pain's intensity. Although it uses a commonly understood concept, it is less sensitive to subtle changes and requires abstract thinking. It is important to verify, however, that the patient can count up to the high end of the scale (Figure 3–2).

Verbal descriptor scales are quick and simple. They require choosing the best descriptor word. It is necessary to remember the words or to have a written form available. Patients must understand the meaning of the words, and assessment may be less accurate as choices are limited. Patients have a tendency to use the middle rather than the ends of category scales, thus altering the decision process and further decreasing possible choices (Figure 3–3).

Regardless of the scale chosen, it is imperative to clarify what level of pain is tolerable or acceptable to the patient. This allows the health care team to set reasonable, reachable goals. Absence of pain is not always possible. Tolerable relief, more activity, and improved eating and sleeping habits may precede reaching the "goal" and should be offered as evidence to the patient that the pain status is improving.

The patient's quality descriptors offer clues about the nociceptive and/or neuropathic components of the pain experience. "Prickly," "shooting," "burning" are terms more likely to be indicative of

None|Annoying|Uncomfortable|Dreadful|Horrible|Agonizing

FIGURE 3–3 *Verbal Descriptor Scale*
Instructions: Choose the word above that best describes how your pain feels right now.

neuropathic pain, whereas "dull," "aching," or "heavy" may describe nociceptive pain. By utilizing the quality descriptors, it may be possible to identify both nociceptive and neuropathic components of the pain experience.

Location is a critical variable. It is best to obtain this information while the pain is actually present, as the accuracy of the patient's report diminishes as the pain recedes. When questioning the location, have the patient point to the source on his or her body, or mark the appropriate anatomic drawing on the assessment tool. Anatomic renderings should include front, back, left side, and right side views of the whole body as well as the right, left, front, and back sides of the head. The majority of assessment tools also include views of both feet. More than one source of pain or the onset of new pain can be identified. Pointing to or marking the location provides specific information that may be missed with verbal description alone. It can also be very helpful to have the patient correlate the anatomic site with quality descriptor words. This allows the clinician the opportunity to clarify his or her understanding of the patient's pain experience.

Awareness of behaviors and/or of interventions that exacerbate or relieve pain contributes valuable diagnostic leads, as well as provides direction for planning analgesic interventions. These queries provide the opportunity to explore behaviors that make the pain worse and identify behaviors, non-pharmacologic and pharmacologic interventions that may significantly reduce the pain level.

The pain's effects on the individual provide a greater understanding of the total pain experience. Knowledge of the pain's effect on functional status, appetite, sleep, cognitive function, emotions/mood, energy levels, sleep, and social relationships allows for more effective planning of therapeutic interventions and assists in identifying the appropriate members of the multidisciplinary team. Studies exploring the correlation between pain intensity and functional status have documented significant correlation between self-report, disease characteristics, and objective functional performance.

OBJECTIVE DATA

Assessment may include vital signs, patient behaviors, and physical appearance as long as they are interpreted in the context of the total pain experience. The patient with chronic pain experiences an adaptation of the autonomic nervous system and may not exhibit any changes in vital signs. As mentioned, the patient in the midst of an acute pain experience is more likely to demonstrate the classic picture of rapid breathing, increased pulse, and increased blood pressure.

This principle of adaptation holds true for behavioral characteristics. One may not see the expected grimacing, crying, and guarding seen in patients experiencing acute pain. Patients may appear to be relaxed or engaged in other activities that are not "appropriate" for a patient in pain. Facial expression may be without affect. For patients who are unable to communicate it is especially important to look for behavioral clues (facial expressions and/or body movements, activity changes such as changing position frequently or sitting stiffly) and question those who know the patient well. The clinician can ask family members and friends whether or not they think the patient has pain and why. If documented pathology clearly indicates the patient *should* have pain, it is reasonable to initiate a trial dose of analgesic and document its effect. If the patient has been on an established regimen, that same regimen should be continued regardless of the patient's ability to verbalize the discomfort. It is also both reasonable and humane to administer an analgesic prophylactically for the noncommunicating patient who is about to undergo a known painful procedure.

Physical appearance also may be affected. Changes in personal grooming habits may occur as the individual pays less attention to personal hygiene and aesthetics and as the focus on pain absorbs available physical and emotional resources.

EFFECTS OF PREVIOUS THERAPY

The effects of previous therapy, such as treatment failures and successes and patient confidence in efficacy, provide a window into the individual's past experiences. A patient's evaluative assessment of prior treatment can eliminate repetitive intervention that is not beneficial or even harmful, as well as call attention to treatment that previously provided relief. Both pharmacologic and nonpharmacologic interventions may be described. For instance, use of a transcutaneous electrical nerve stimulation (TENS) unit for an identified trial period with no effect may eliminate that choice; successful intervention with an opioid analgesic at a certain dosage may again be successful if the dosage is increased. Patient confidence is an essential assessment factor. A firm belief or disbelief in the efficacy of an intervention can predispose that intervention to success or failure.

CURRENT ANALGESIC THERAPY

Current medications, dosages, doses required per day, route, and efficacy need to be evaluated. Side effects of therapy and their management should be queried as well. Cognitive/behavioral, physical therapy modalities, other nonpharmacologic interventions, and any alternative therapies the patient is currently using should be reviewed.

CULTURAL AND RELIGIOUS VARIABLES

Cultural and religious perspectives superimpose behaviors, viewpoints, and convictions integral to the individual. This cultural/religious grid functions as an experiential filter that determines the person's response to pain and planned interventions. Cultural expectations affect pain behaviors, and lack of understanding of those expectations may result in inaccurate assessment. For example, if cultural expectations demand a stoic demeanor even in the presence of severe pain, the patient's calm affect and denial of pain may not accurately reflect the pain's intensity.

The meaning of the pain can have a significant impact on treatment. For instance, if an individual believes that the disease and subsequent pain is a well-deserved punishment from a higher being or is to be accepted as inevitable or as a predetermined learning experience, accurate self-report and compliance with therapy can be compromised. For some patients pain may have significant value. It may be a reminder that they are still alive or may serve to draw attention to themselves as individuals. For others it may serve only as a reminder that they have a life-threatening or terminal illness. It is important to clarify the fear and/or anxiety that the pain experience provokes so that physiologic and psychologic interventions can be identified and implemented.

PSYCHOSOCIAL MODIFIERS

Awareness of personal/family dynamics and concurrent stressors allows greater insight into the individual's response to pain. Personality characteristics define behavior patterns. Observation of family interaction may provide information the health care team can use to intervene more successfully. As pain can be an energy-draining experience, the presence of concurrent stressors can further compromise energy reserves and interfere with successful treatment.

The frequency of the assessment is determined by the severity of the pain and/or the stability of analgesic relief. Like vital signs, pain needs more frequent assessment when there is an unresolved problem. Acute, unrelieved pain requires frequent assessment until acceptable control is achieved (e.g., postoperative patients should be assessed hourly until a stable dosage and schedule is determined). Chronic pain that is well controlled may be assessed less frequently. When pain is escalating, ongoing assessment is required to evaluate the efficacy of interventions.

A baseline assessment is made easier by a standardized format that incorporates anatomic charts for indicating pain sites and a pain intensity scale that documents initial measurement. Ongoing monitoring allows for tracking of changes in the pain over time and response to treatment. Nursing monitoring tools include *flow sheets,* which can be used to track pain and related symptoms such as nausea or sedation, and *graphic records of pain intensity,* which, when charted alongside vital signs patterns, make pain more readily visible and objective. A *diary* is particularly useful for outpatients. It allows for a longer time between assessments. It has the advantage of providing a more accurate picture of the nature of the pain in the patient's own surroundings or under more usual circumstances. It also may be used to track other symptoms.

A thorough and accurate diagnostic assessment is vital to provide the patient the most effective interventions possible. When well done, therapeutic interventions are far more likely to have a positive effect. Collaborative efforts from other health team members in providing ongoing assessment afford the patient the necessary monitoring and follow-up on which excellence in pain relief is predicated.

BIBLIOGRAPHY

Bonica, J.J., & Loeser, J.D. (1990). Medical evaluation of the patient with pain. In J.J. Bonica (Ed.), *The management of pain* (2nd ed.), pp. 563–579. Philadelphia: Lea & Febiger.

Chapman, C.R., & Syrjala, K.L. (1990). Measurement of pain. In J.J. Bonica (Ed.), *The management of pain* (2nd ed)., pp. 580–594. Philadelphia: Lea & Febiger.

Daut, R.L., Cleeland, C.S., & Flanery, R.C. (1983). Development of the Wisconsin brief pain questionnaire to assess pain in cancer and other diseases. *Pain, 17,* 197–210.

Fishman, B., et al. (1986). The Memorial Pain Assessment Card: A valid instrument for evaluation of cancer pain (abstr). *American Journal of Clinical Oncology, 5,* 239.

Hathaway, S.R., & McKinley, J.C. (1967). *The Minnesota Multiphasic Personality Inventory manual.* New York: Psychological Corporation.

Helmes, E.H. (1994). What types of useful information do the MMPI and MMPI-2 provide on patients with chronic pain? *APS Bulletin, 4*(1), 1–2, 5.

Keller, L.S., & Butcher, J.N. (1991). *Assessment of chronic pain patients with the MMPI-2.* (p. 362). Minneapolis: The University of Minnesota Press.

McCaffery, J. (1979). *Nursing management of the patient with pain.* New York: Lippincott.

McCaffery, M., & Beebe, A. (1989). Assessment. In *Pain. Clinical manual for nursing practice* (pp. 6–33). St. Louis: Mosby.

Melzack, R. (1975). The McGill pain questionnaire: Major properties and scoring methods. *Pain, 1,* 275–279.

Melzack, R. (1987). The short-form McGill pain questionnaire. *Pain, 30,* 191–197.

Morey, L.C. (1991). *Personality Assessment Inventory professional manual.* Odessa, FL: Psychological Assessment Resources.

Pincus, T., Callahan, L.F., Bradley, L.A., Vaugh, W.K., & Wolfe, F. (1986). Elevated MMPI scores for hypochondriasis, depression, and hysteria in patients with rheumatoid arthritis reflect disease rather than psychological status. *Arthritis and Rheumatitis, 29,* 1456–1466.

Turner, J.A., & Romano, J.M. (1990). Psychologic and psychosocial evaluation. In J.J. Bonica (Ed.), *The management of pain* (2nd ed.), pp. 595–609. Philadelphia: Lea & Febiger.

4
Pharmacology

Nonopioid, opioid, and atypical **analgesic** preparations are used singly and in combination to treat both acute and chronic pain conditions. They may be used concurrently with nonpharmacologic modalities as well as in combination with anesthetic procedures. Although the primary goal of treatment should be to address the underlying etiology of the pain, analgesics may be used to relieve symptoms, such as pain and inflammation, on a short-term or long-term basis. They may be prescribed on an as-needed or scheduled basis depending on the nature and intensity of the pain. Chronic pain conditions, both malignant and nonmalignant, may require scheduled dosing for extended periods or even over the lifetime.

Chapter 2 briefly reviewed the anatomy and physiology particular to the transmission of the pain signal and identified pharmacologic agents that interfere with or modulate that transmission. Although nonopioid analgesics primarily relieve pain at the peripheral nervous system level by interfering with prostaglandin synthesis and opioid analgesics work primarily at the central nervous system (CNS) level by attaching to opioid receptors, atypical (sometimes referred to as adjuvant) analgesics demonstrate varied mechanisms of action.

The atypical analgesics encompass a diverse body of drugs. Even though they are clearly able to provide analgesic relief in specific patient populations, they should not be considered primary analgesics as they do not possess the same efficacy as the opioids. In some chronic nonmalignant pain syndromes (e.g., diabetic neuropathy), they may be prescribed as primary treatment with opioid analgesics as secondary agents. In other chronic pain syndromes (e.g., a malignancy that has infiltrated part of the nervous system), the opioid analgesic will be prescribed as the primary agent and the atypical analgesic will serve in an adjuvant capacity. In addition to providing analgesia for specific types of pain, atypical analgesics are used to potentiate the analgesic effects of the opioids and treat associated symptoms that exacerbate pain. Corticosteroids, tricyclic antidepressants, anticonvulsants, local anesthetics, antiarrhythmics, and benzodiazepines are primary examples and are discussed in more detail in the latter part of this chapter.

NONOPIOID ANALGESICS

Nonopioid analgesics include acetaminophen (e.g., Tylenol®) and the nonsteroidal antiinflammatory agents (NSAIDs), such as ibuprofen (Motrin®), salsalate (Disalcid®), and naproxen (Naproxyn®). Aspirin is considered to be an NSAID because of its powerful anti-inflammatory effects. Acetaminophen does not have anti-inflammatory properties, so it is excluded from the NSAID classification. It is unclear exactly how acetaminophen provides analgesic relief, although it is hypothesized that it works in a similar manner to the NSAIDs. Their primary mechanism of action centers on inhibiting prostaglandin synthesis at the peripheral nervous system level, thereby inhibiting the ability of prostaglandins to sensitize nerve endings to pain-producing stimuli. There is, however, increasing evidence that they also may have some activity at the CNS level. Although they are very different structurally, the nonopioids share analgesic, antipyretic, anti-inflammatory, and antiplatelet properties to different degrees. Typical indications include varied types of acute and/or chronic pain conditions: headache, arthritis, mild postoperative or traumatic discomfort, toothache, orthopedic injuries, low-back pain, menstrual pain, and mild to moderate cancer pain (Table 4–1). Both acetaminophen and aspirin can be very useful, but their maximum recommended daily doses may not offer enough analgesic relief for some chronic nonmalignant pain syndromes. As is true for the NSAIDs, they are contraindicated in specific patient populations.

Text continued on page 45

TABLE 4–1 *Nonopioid Treatment Variables*

Advantages	Disadvantages
Excellent analgesia for mild to moderate pain	Efficacy limited to mild to moderate pain
No dependence liability/tolerance development	Varied patient responses
Most opioid side effects are absent	Ceiling effect (higher dosage does not increase analgesia)
Equianalgesic to many oral weak opioids	Longer half-lives of many can produce toxicity in patients who are aged or have severe renal or hepatic dysfunction
Analgesic dosage may be lower than anti-inflammatory dosage	Appreciable toxicity with chronic use: bleeding tendencies (interfere with platelet aggregation); gastrointestinal intolerance and ulcerations: cytoprotective mechanism of prostaglandins is interrupted by NSAIDs and aspirin; renal insufficiency: prostaglandins have an important role in maintaining renal blood flow
Easier to obtain than opioid analgesics: many are available over the counter and can be quite inexpensive	Routes of administration limited
	Full benefit occurs after a week or more
	Effects underrated: may not be used appropriately

TABLE 4-2 *Selected Nonopioid Analgesics*

Chemical Class	Generic/ Trade Name	Dosing Interval (Hours)	Average Dose	Maximum Recommended Dose (mg/day)	Equianalgesic Dose		Comments	Clinical Considerations
Para-aminophenol derivatives	Acetaminophen (Tylenol®)	4–6	325–1000 mg q4-6h	4,000	Oral agents		Hepatic toxicity secondary to overdosage	Monitor daily cumulative dosage, being sure to account for that found in combination analgesics.
					Acetaminophen	650 mg	Not anti-inflammatory, therefore not recommended as coanalgesic for bone pain	May be given with other NSAIDs. May serve as effective coanalgesic in patients who are thrombocytopenic. As it is available in suppositories, tablets, capsules, and oral solution, alternative routes may be chosen for the patient who has difficulty swallowing. Potential hepatotoxicity increased by carbamazepine (Tegretol®)
					Aspirin	650 mg		
					Codeine	32 mg	Lacks GI and platelet toxicity	
					Hydrocodone	5 mg	Administration to patients with chronic alcoholism or liver disease increases risk for hepatotoxicity	
					Meperidine	50 mg		
					Propoxyphene napsylate	100 mg		

40

Class	Drug	Half-life (h)	Dose	Maximum dose (mg)	Comparison	Pharmacology	Clinical comments
Salicylates Acetylated	Aspirin	4–6	325–650 mg q4h	4,000		Potent inhibitor of prostaglandin synthesis Inhibits platelet aggregation, a property associated with the acetyl group; irreversible for the life of the platelet May decrease NSAID serum concentration; avoid concomitant use	Monitor for GI intolerance, ulceration, and bleeding Use cautiously in patients with chronic renal insufficiency, gastric ulcers, peptic ulcers, or bleeding tendencies Assess patient usage of over-the-counter medications. May contain aspirin. Availability in rectal form makes it suitable for patients unable to swallow Do not use in children <12 with possible viral illness
Nonacetylated	Diflunisal (Dolobid®)	8–12	1,000 mg ×1 500 then 500 mg q8–12h	1500 mg	1000 mg of Dolobid is comparable to 600 mg acetaminophen with 60 mg codeine	Less GI intolerance and bleeding than with aspirin No effect on platelet aggregation Potent anti-inflammatory effects	Diflunisal is less likely to reduce fever than other NSAIDs. May be useful when monitoring temperatures in the neutropenic patient. Limited effect on platelet aggregation advantageous for the thrombocytopenic patient. Twice daily dosing an advantage for patients on multiple medications.
	Choline magnesium trisalicylate (Trilisate®)	12	1,000–1,500 mg q12h	2,000–3,000			

Table continued on following page

TABLE 4-2 *Selected Nonopioid Analgesics (Continued)*

Chemical Class	Generic/ Trade Name	Dosing Interval (Hours)	Average Dose	Maximum Recommended Dose (mg/day)	Equianalgesic Dose	Comments	Clinical Considerations
	Salsalate (Disalcid®)	8–12	1,500 mg x 1 1,000 mg q8–12h	2,000–3,000			*Choline magnesium trisalicylate* is available in liquid form for patients who have difficulty swallowing
Propionic acid derivatives	Ibuprofen (Advil®, Motrin®, Nuprin®)	4–6	200–400 q4–6h	2,400	Superior at 200 mg to 650 mg aspirin	Available over-the-counter. Better tolerated than aspirin with less intense GI side effects. Lower incidence of hepatotoxic effects than with aspirin or other NSAIDs	*Ibuprofen* and *naproxen* are available in suspension form for patients who have difficulty swallowing Assess and carefully monitor patients concurrently on ibuprofen and corticosteroids; there is an increased risk of GI toxicity
	Naproxen (Naprosyn®)	6–8	500 mg x 1 250 mg q6–8h	1,250		Long-term efficacy and safety at recommended dos-	Monitor patients on high doses bi-monthly: stool guiac, liver function tests,

Class	Drug	Half-life (h)	Dose	Max (mg)	Equivalence	Comments
	Naproxen Sodium (Anaprox®, Aleve®)	6–8	550 mg × 1 275 mg q6–8h	1,375	275 mg = 650 mg aspirin	blood urea nitrogen, creatinine, urinalysis ages is unknown. Use cautiously in selected patients.
	Fenoprofen (Nalfon®)	4–6	200 mg q4–6h	800		
	Ketoprofen (Orudis®)	6–8	25–75 mg q6–8h	300		
Acetic acids	Indomethacin (Indocin®)	6–12	25–50 mg q6–12	100–200		Potent inhibitor of prostaglandin synthesis—may exert greater analgesic and anti-inflammatory effect than aspirin Serious GI toxicity Rectal route, although convenient for some patients, may cause irritation, mucosal inflammation, or necrosis with bleeding Assess patient for history of GI lesions. *Indomethacin* is not appropriate for those patients Less renal toxicity than other NSAIDs (Clinoril)
	Tolmetin (Tolectin®)	6–8	200–600 mg q6–8h	1,800		
	Sulindac (Clinoril®)	12	150–200 mg q12h	400		
	Diclofenac Sodium (Voltaren®)	6–8	50 mg q8h	200		

Table continued on following page

43

TABLE 4-2 *Selected Nonopioid Analgesics (Continued)*

CHEMICAL CLASS	GENERIC/ TRADE NAME	DOSING INTERVAL (HOURS)	AVERAGE DOSE	MAXIMUM RECOMMENDED DOSE (MG/DAY)	EQUIANALGESIC DOSE	COMMENTS	CLINICAL CONSIDERATIONS
	Ketorolac (Toradol®)	6	30-60 mg IM/IV × 1 15-30 mg IM/IV q6h	120	30-60 mg comparable to 6-12 mg IM morphine sulfate	No experience with chronic administration. Analgesic effect may be greater than antiinflammatory effect.	May be given IV or IM. Uncomfortable when given IM Peak analgesic effects occur 1-2 hours after administration. Assess efficacy at this time. Not to be administered for more than 5 days Oral regimen should be discontinued after 14 days
Oxicams	Piroxicam (Feldene®)	24	10 mg PO q4-6h 20 mg	40 40		Administration of 40 mg >3 weeks is associated with a high incidence of peptic ulcer disease	Daily dosing is convenient for patients on multiple medications

Treatment Guidelines

The following treatment guidelines are useful when choosing a nonopioid analgesic:

1. *Assess risks and benefits.* Nonopioid drugs are not benign substances and carry their own side effect profiles. They are contraindicated in identified patient populations. Those patients with a history of chronic renal disease, gastrointestinal (GI) ulcerations or bleeding, and blood dyscrasias or reduced platelet counts may be harmed by these analgesics. See Table 4–2 for more details.

2. *Titrate the dosage.* Start with a low dosage to ascertain patient reaction and then increase gradually. Lack of efficacy may be secondary to the specific drug or the dosage. Administer at the maximally tolerated dosage for 1 to 2 weeks to properly evaluate efficacy.

3. *Choose a different NSAID if the current one is ineffective.* Assuming that the pain status is unchanged and relief is inadequate at the maximally tolerated dose for a period of 1 to 2 weeks, select another with a different chemical structure. The second drug may interfere with prostaglandin synthesis in a different way and thus have more efficacy. When trialing the NSAIDs, change once or twice to alternative agents. If sufficient relief at the maximally tolerated dosage is not obtained, an opioid analgesic may be required.

4. *Do not combine NSAIDs.* This includes aspirin. There is an increased risk of gastric and renal toxicity. Acetaminophen is an exception and may be used in combination with NSAIDs.

5. *Differentiate analgesic versus anti-inflammatory effects.* An effective dose should provide analgesia within 2 hours with the analgesic dosage typically lower than the anti-inflammatory dosage. Maximal anti-inflammatory effects occur later as the serum level accumulates. Regular dosing for at least a week may provide increased pain relief.

6. *Tailor the analgesic to the severity of the pain.* When the nonopioids no longer provide pain relief, it may be necessary to add an opioid analgesic. Nonopioids may be used in conjunction with an opioid analgesic. This combination addresses the pain at both the peripheral and central nervous system levels and may provide superior analgesic relief. Dosing the patient with an opioid and nonopioid simultaneously may provide not only increased relief but also increased duration of effect. If using a nonopioid/opioid compound (e.g., Percocet®, Vicodin®, Darvocet®) monitor the daily dosage of the nonopioid so that the recommended cumulative daily dose is not exceeded.

OPIOID ANALGESICS

Opioid analgesics are a group of morphinelike formulations whose properties are primarily analgesic. They interact with multiple kinds of opioid receptors to produce analgesia at the spinal and supraspinal levels. Although there is increasing evidence that they also demonstrate activity at the peripheral level, at present the majority of activity is identified at the CNS level. See Chapter 2 for a more detailed discussion of opioid receptor activity.

Opioid analgesics are used to manage moderate to severe acute pain; recurrent acute pain (i.e., sickle cell disease crisis); prolonged time-limited pain (e.g., cancer pain, burn pain); immediate relief of sudden and severe pain (e.g., renal colic, trauma); immediate, very brief, and reversible relief of moderate to severe pain (e.g., cystoscopy performed with IV opioids and reversed with naloxone [Narcan®] at the end of the procedure); and for selected patients with chronic nonmalignant pain who do not benefit from other analgesic methods but can function on a stabilized dose of opioid analgesic (e.g., severe low-back pain).

Opioid analgesics used to treat mild to moderate pain (e.g., codeine, hydrocodone, oxycodone, propoxyphene) are more likely to have a ceiling effect evidenced by inadequate analgesia with dose-limiting side effects. They often are compounded in fixed-ratio combinations with nonopioid analgesics, which limits the maximum 24-hour recommended dosage and precludes further analgesic relief. Examples include Tylenol #3®, Tylenol #4®, Vicodin®, Roxicodone®, Percocet®, Percodan®, Darvocet®, and Darvocet N-100®.

Opioid analgesics used to treat moderate to severe pain (e.g., fentanyl [Duragesic®], hydromorphone [Dilaudid®], levorphanol [Levo-Dromoran®], methadone [Dolophine®], and morphine) are widely available as noncompounded agents in multiple formulations. Parenteral, intraspinal, oral, sublingual, rectal, and transdermal preparations render them available to patients at varying stages of the disease continuum and at varying levels of cooperation and consciousness. Their onset and duration of action are known, and thus their efficacy can be evaluated early on in the therapeutic course.

As stated, opioids may be used to treat moderate to severe nociceptive pain, but their efficacy in treating pain of neuropathic origin is a matter of controversy. Patients experiencing neuropathic pain syndromes and those with pain of unclear etiology seem less likely to receive adequate analgesia from opioid doses that are efficacious in patients with nociceptive pain. Portenoy, Foley, and Inturrisi (1990) argue for a more explicit definition and characteristics of opioid responsiveness. Significant patient variance has led to the persuasive clinical recommendation that opioid responsiveness be evaluated by (1) the response to a range of doses; (2) the degree of analgesia obtained; and (3) setting the endpoint at either analgesia or unmanageable side effects. Escalating dosage often is handicapped by the development of side effects that are treatable (Table 4–3). Aggressive management of these side effects may allow further escalation of the dose with resultant analgesia.

Both patient-related and pain-related factors are implicated in the issue of opioid responsiveness. Patients may be inclined to opioid-induced side effects because of pharmacokinetic factors (individual differ-

TABLE 4–3 *Considerations for Opioid Usage*

ADVANTAGES	DISADVANTAGES
Excellent analgesia for moderate to severe pain	Side effect profiles include nausea/vomiting, constipation, central nervous system activity
Benefit realized relatively quickly	Tolerance to analgesic effects can develop with extended use
No ceiling effect: increased dosage provides increased analgesia	Dependence liability
Available in multiple forms: parenteral, intraspinal, oral, sublingual, rectal, transdermal; immediate and controlled release	Patient/health care provider fear/reluctance to use opioids

ences in metabolism) or pharmacodynamic factors, although the most common factor is probably advanced age. Significant psychologic distress may influence patient response to opioids by the effect of emotional disturbance on the pain complaint. Prior exposure to significant doses of opioids with the accompanying development of tolerance does not automatically reduce opioid responsiveness, but these patients do require significant incremental increases to achieve greater pain relief. The use of a small analgesic dose would most likely provide no effect and lead to the mistaken conclusion of opioid unresponsiveness.

The choice of drug may be a factor in opioid responsiveness. Clinical experience has demonstrated that patients can respond poorly and have unmanageable side effects on one opioid but have a significantly different experience when switched to another. This repudiates the idea that any one opioid is intrinsically more effective. When dose escalation with any opioid yields intolerable and unmanageable side effects with or without adequate analgesia, another opioid should be trialed.

Pain-related factors have been a primary focal point when examining opioid responsiveness. Pains of rapid onset or those that progress rapidly may be relatively more difficult to control with opioids than pain with other profiles. This may be related to the inability to deliver enough drug quickly enough to have a significant analgesic effect. Neuropathic pain, which follows injury to the peripheral or central nervous system, involves multiple mechanisms in signal transmission. As this type of pain seems to involve different mechanisms from the nociceptive pathway, opioid responsiveness may differ. These patients require greater analgesic doses than those with nociceptive pain and thus could be seen as relatively less responsive. There is no definitive answer as to why this occurs, but one hypothesis focuses on the relation of neuropathic pain to activity in usually non-nociceptive large myelinated afferent nerve fibers. Because opioids are known to be effective by interfering with nociceptive activity in the dorsal horn, these other mechanisms may cause the pain to be less responsive. Because it has been demonstrated that neuropathic pain is relatively less responsive to opioid analgesics (i.e., a greater dosage is required to provide analgesia), it can be concluded that responsiveness is a continuum and that neuropathic mechanisms may be one of the factors associated with a diminished clinical response. That analysis supports the clinical conclusion that a trial of opioid therapy in patients with significant pain should not be withheld or limited on the basis of inferred pathophysiology alone.

The same opioid receptors at the CNS level that mediate analgesia also mediate other physiologic phenomena. Tolerance to the analgesic effects of opioids is at least partially mediated by the interaction of opioids with the mu receptors. There is some evidence that each of the different receptor subtypes is under independent genetic control, so that the interaction between a particular drug and particular receptor may vary. Clinical observations that tolerance develops to different opioids at different rates may be partially explained by this rationale. Thus it stands to reason that a change in opioid analgesics could result in incomplete cross-tolerance and clinically provide increased analgesia with a lesser equianalgesic dosage.

Patients who are on significant and escalating doses of opioid analgesics are usually those who have disease progression and subsequent progression of the pain state. In those instances it is difficult to distinguish between tolerance and the analgesic requirements of disease progression. This is common in the oncology patient population.

Tolerance develops more rapidly when opioids are administered parenterally than when they are administered orally or rectally. Early indications are decreased duration of analgesic effect, which is treated clinically by an increase in the analgesic dosage or change in the schedule. In summary, strategies for delaying tolerance include: (1) using a multidrug regimen that includes analgesics with different mechanisms of action (e.g., nonopioids and opioids) to reduce overall opioid dosage; (2) relying on nonparenteral routes whenever possible; and (3) changing to an alternative opioid when dosage is escalating rapidly.

Physical dependence is primarily mediated by the mu receptors with some help from the kappa receptors. When opioid intervention is discontinued at too rapid a pace after significant previous exposure, the withdrawal syndrome may include yawning, lacrimation, frequent sneezing, agitation, tremors, insomnia, fever, tachycardia, and other signs of hyperexcitability of the sympathetic nervous system. The characteristics and time of onset may vary. Strategies to forestall acute withdrawal in patients whose pain is diminished focus on incremental decreases in the opioid dose. The dose should be decreased by 25% to 50% each day depending on the degree to which the pain has subsided and the need for additional doses for breakthrough pain. Patients without pain whose doses are being tapered should be given at least 25% of their previous day's doses to prevent physical withdrawal.

Fear of respiratory depression often is cited as the reason for cautious dosing when using opioid analgesics. Respiratory depression can occur via direct effect on the chemoreceptors of the respiratory center in the brainstem. Maximal depression occurs within 5 to 10 minutes after intravenous administration, 30 minutes after intramuscular administration, and 90 minutes after subcutaneous administration. As pain, analgesic, sedative, and respiratory depression thresholds are sequential, careful titration and monitoring can prevent this problem in most instances. Respiratory depression is unusual in the patient who has been chronically exposed to opioids and can more often be attributed to coexisting pathophysiology.

Depressive effects on the CNS may include heaviness in the extremities, drowsiness, mood changes, including euphoria, mental clouding, and sedation. Tolerance to the sedative effects of appropriate doses usually develops within 1 to 3 days. The use of opioid-sparing, nonsedating drugs used in combination with the opioids can also help. Persistent sedation can be reduced with caffeine or methylphenidate (Ritalin®).

If a patient suffers intolerable and unmanageable confusion when on an opioid analgesic regimen, it is appropriate to switch to another opioid even if it is not conclusive that the opioid is the culprit. Other physiologic factors can cause confusion, so the clinical picture may be somewhat muddy. If the confusion resolves, the problem is solved. Persistent confusion may dissipate with haloperidol (Haldol®) administration.

High parenteral doses of opioids may stimulate the CNS and cause excitation and seizures. Meperidine (Demerol®) is a well-known culprit. When metabolized, it is transformed to normeperidine, which accumulates with repetitive dosing and can lead to seizures. Any of the opioids, when administered in significant doses, can cause myoclonus, a twitching or clonic spasm of a muscle or group of muscles. Myoclonic jerks can be treated with clonazepam (Klonopin®), an anticonvulsant, or one of the well-known muscle relaxants.

Opioids can significantly affect the GI tract. A decrease in secretions and peristalsis produces constipation. Tolerance to the constipating effects does not develop, and this problem must be addressed as long as the patient remains on analgesic therapy. There are numerous bowel regimens currently in use that can be tailored to patient specifications. The primary principle is to titrate by using a stepped approach. Begin with a stool softener and/or gentle laxative (e.g., Colace®, Peri-colace®, Senekot®, Senekot-S®). If there are no results within 48 hours, add a stimulant (e.g., Dulcolax®), lactulose, or milk of magnesia. If results do not follow, perform a rectal examination to rule out impaction and try a Dulcolax® suppository, magnesium citrate, or an enema. If the patient is impacted, manual disimpaction preceded by a softening agent (glycerin suppository or mineral oil retention enema) may be necessary. It is imperative to control constipation as it can cause significant distress.

Direct stimulation of the chemoreceptor trigger zone (CTZ) can produce nausea and vomiting. This emetogenic effect, generally observed only with initial doses, can be controlled with an antiemetic agent that may be slowly tapered off over the course of initial therapy. Centrally acting antiemetics such as prochlorperazine (Compazine®), metoclopramide (Reglan®), or droperidol (Inapsine®) may be used. If the nausea/vomiting is unmanageable even with aggressive therapy, it is appropriate to choose another opioid analgesic. The nausea/vomiting may not occur with the second choice.

Urinary effects include bladder spasm and urgency or conversely, difficulty in urination and urinary retention. Retention often occurs at the initiation of therapy, but tolerance to this side effect usually develops within days to weeks. If output is not secondary to other identifiable causes, oxybutytnin (Ditropan®) may be trialed.

Treatment Guidelines

The following treatment guidelines should be kept in mind when using opioid analgesics:

1. Treatment of pain begins by treating the underlying etiology. Nonopioids and the atypi-

cal analgesics may follow. If an opioid is to be used, begin with the mildest opioid preparation that controls the pain. The use of nonopioids and atypical analgesics may increase the analgesic effect and provide an opioid dose-sparing effect.

2. When a fixed-ratio combination nonopioid/opioid analgesic does not provide relief at the maximum recommended daily dosage, it may be necessary to alter the opioid regimen by changing to another opioid or adding another opioid preparation to the current regimen (e.g., maximum daily recommended dose of Percocet® may be supplemented by oxycodone tablets).

3. When opioids are used on a chronic or long-term basis, the pure agonist opioids (codeine, hydrocodone, oxycodone, morphine, hydromorphone, methadone, levorphanol, and fentanyl) should be used. Although it is an opioid agonist, meperidine (Demerol®) is not recommended for chronic use because the accumulation of its active metabolite, normeperidine, can cause CNS excitatory effects.

4. Cautiously use the agonist-antagonist opioids pentazocine (Talwin®), nalbuphine (Nubain®), butorphanol (Stadol®), and buprenorphine (Buprenex®) for chronic dosing. Although they have a ceiling effect for respiratory depression and are less likely to produce tolerance, there is significant incidence of psychotomimetic effects. They should not be administered simultaneously with opioid analgesics as they will function in an antagonist capacity and displace the opioid from the mu receptor.

5. When initiating any opioid therapy, assess the patient thoroughly and frequently. Those patients who are opioid-naive require careful observation as the dosage is titrated. Failure to monitor may lead to under- or overdosage.

6. Utilize opioid equianalgesic knowledge to make decisions when changing the opioid preparation or route of delivery. See Tables 4–4 and 4–5.

TABLE 4–4 *Equianalgesic Chart: Simplified Equianalgesia for Commonly Prescribed Oral Analgesics*

TRADE NAME (GENERIC) ORAL MEDICATION	EQUAL TO ORAL MORPHINE (MG)	EQUAL TO IM/IV MORPHINE (MG)
Dilaudid® (hydromorphone) 1 mg	4	1.3
Codeine 30 mg	4.5	1.5
Darvon® (propoxyphene hydrochloride) 65 mg or Darvocet N 50® (propoxyphene napsylate + 325 mg acetaminophen) or Demerol® (meperidine) 50 mg	4.5	1.6
Tylenol #3® (30 mg codeine + 300 mg acetaminophen) or Percocet® (oxycodone 5 mg + 325 mg acetaminophen) or Percodan® (oxycodone 5 mg + 325 mg aspirin)	7.2	2.4
Vicodin® (hydrocodone 5 mg + 500 mg acetaminophen) or Tylox® (oxycodone 5 mg + 500 mg acetaminophen) or Darvocet N 100® (propoxyphene napsylate 100 mg + 600 mg acetaminophen)	9	3
Dolophine® (methadone) 10 mg	15	5
Tylenol® (acetaminophen) 325 mg	2.7	0.9
Tylenol Extra Strength® (acetaminophen) 500 mg	4	1.3
Tylenol #4® (60 mg codeine + 300 mg acetaminophen)	11.7	3.9

Table continued on page 55

TABLE 4–4 *Equianalgesic Chart: Simplified Equianalgesia for Commonly Prescribed Oral Analgesics (Continued)*

Trade Name (Generic) Oral Medication	Equal to Oral Morphine (mg)	Equal to IM/IV Morphine (mg)
Duragesic® patch (transdermal fentanyl): based on 25-µg patch applied every 3 days = 50 mg oral morphine every 25 hours or divided into 6 doses = 8.3 mg)	8.3	2.77

Adapted with permission from Betty Ferrell, Ph.D., F.A.A.N., City of Hope National Medical Center. Based on published equianalgesic data.

7. Prescribe as needed or scheduled dosing based on the known half-life of the drug. Scheduling intervals that exceed the opioid's duration of effect set the patient up for inadequate relief.

8. When using opioids on a chronic basis, assess for tolerance (stable pain level requiring increased opioid dosage). When opioids are used in the management of chronic nonmalignant pain, they are generally recommended for pain that is resistant to curative interventions, anesthetic procedures, nonpharmacologic interventions, and nonopioid preparations. See Chapter 9 for further considerations.

9. Patients receiving chronic opioid therapy usually develop tolerance to the respiratory depressant effects of the drugs. The administration of opioid antagonists, such as naloxone, should be approached cautiously. Patients who are opioid tolerant demonstrate great sensitivity to the effects of antagonist drugs. If it is essential to treat respiratory depression, the naloxone should be diluted (0.4 mg in 10 ml of saline) and

Text continued on page 63

TABLE 4-5 *Selected Opioid Analgesics*

GENERIC NAME	EQUANALGESIC DOSE (STANDARD OF COMPARISON 10 MG IM MORPHINE)	APPROXIMATE HALF-LIFE (HOURS)	DOSING INTERVAL (HOURS)	COMMENTS	CLINICAL CONSIDERATIONS
Mild to moderate pain				Analgesic effect due to conversion to morphine No advantage over morphine when administered parenterally	Constipation and nausea can be significant; increased incidence of side effects at dosages >1.5 mg/kg At least 60 mg needed to provide increased analgesia over 650 mg aspirin or 650 mg acetaminophen.
Codeine (Tylenol #3®, Tylenol #4®)	130 mg IM 200 mg PO	3–4	3–4	Found frequently in combination with nonopioid analgesics	Most patients cannot tolerate this dosage When administered concurrently with cimetidine (Tagamet®) or fluoxetine (Prozac®), codeine may not be converted into morphine, and therefore offer little, if any, analgesic relief

Oxycodone (Percocet®, Percodan®, Roxicet®)	30 mg PO	2–3	3–4	Found frequently in combination with nonopioid analgesics (aspirin and acetaminophen)	While found in combination with aspirin or acetaminophen, it is also available as a single agent that allows an increase in dosage without the dose-limiting toxicity of the nonopioid. However, the 5-mg tablet is inconvenient at higher doses. If administered in fixed dosage ratio, monitor for the cumulative dosage of the nonopioid
Controlled-Release Oxycodone (Oxycontin®)	30 mg PO		2–3		The controlled-release form, Oxycontin®, is available in 10-, 20-, and 40-mg sizes, which allows for ease of dosing and serves as an alternative for controlled-release morphine
Meperidine (Demerol®)	100 mg IM 300 mg PO		2–3	Short acting; transformed to normeperidine, a toxic metabolite that accumu-	The administration of naloxone (Narcan®) to patients with normeperidine-in-

Table continued on following page

TABLE 4-5 *Selected Opioid Analgesics* (Continued)

GENERIC NAME	EQUIANALGESIC DOSE (STANDARD OF COMPARISON) 10 MG IM MORPHINE)	APPROXIMATE HALF-LIFE (HOURS)	DOSING INTERVAL (HOURS)	COMMENTS	CLINICAL CONSIDERATIONS
				lates with repetitive dosing, causing CNS excitation Avoid in patients with impaired renal function or concurrent monoamine oxidase inhibitors	duced CNS toxicity may precipitate seizures by interfering with the CNS-depressant effects of meperidine and allowing the convulsant effects of normeperidine to prevail
Propoxyphene (Darvon®, Darvocet®)	NA	12	3–6	Toxic metabolite norpropoxyphene accumulates with repetitive dosing Often combined in fixed dosage ratio with nonopioids	Not recommended for routine use because of long half-life and risk of accumulation of norpropoxyphene, a toxic metabolite
Moderate to severe pain					
Morphine	10 mg IM, 30–60 mg PO	3–4	3–4	Standard of comparison for opioid analgesics Multiple routes available Accumulation of morphine-6-glucuronide, an active	Availability of oral (tablet, controlled-release, and elixir) and rectal formulations often precludes the use of more inva-

Controlled-release morphine (MS Contin®, Oramorph®)	30–60 mg PO	2–3	8–12	metabolite, can be toxic in patients with mild renal insufficiency; may cause chronic nausea and confusion
				The controlled-release form allows the patient to be less dependent on the medication schedule
				"Gold standard" to manage cancer pain, but other equally efficacious opioids may be used for those patients intolerant of morphine
Hydromorphone (Dilaudid®)	1.5 mg IM 7.5 mg PO	2–4	3–4	Has a short half-life and quick onset of action
				Essentially equal to morphine at equianalgesic doses
				Six times as soluble in aqueous solutions as morphine and four times as potent. It is available in high-concentration parenteral form, which allows lower volumes when administered intravenously or subcutaneously via a patient-controlled analgesia device

Table continued on following page

TABLE 4-5 *Selected Opioid Analgesics* (Continued)

Generic Name	Equianalgesic Dose (Standard of comparison 10 mg IM Morphine)	Approximate Half-Life (hours)	Dosing Interval (hours)	Comments	Clinical Considerations
Levorphanol (Levodromoran®)	2 mg IM 4 mg PO	12–16	6–8	Highly potent synthetic opioid that produces analgesia equal to morphine	The high oral/parenteral ratio makes the oral route inconvenient at high doses Titration of the dosage requires careful observation. The long half-life allows the possibility of excessive drug accumulation Seems to cause less nausea/vomiting than morphine
Methadone (Dolophine®)	10 mg IM 20 mg PO	15–30	6–8	When titrating the initial dose, administer modest amounts for up to a week; the maximum effect is not observed until 4–7 days after initiation of therapy	Duration of analgesic effect is shorter than half-life Frequent dose escalations and short dose intervals will lead to increasing accumulation, which may result in toxic serum levels

Fentanyl (Sublimaze®)	100 µg	3.5	½–1	Synthetic opioid that is approximately 75 times more potent than morphine. Not routinely used intravenously in the acute care or outpatient setting. Routinely used for analgesia and anesthesia in the operating suite	The onset of action is almost immediate when administered intravenously, but the maximal analgesic and respiratory depressant effects may not be evident for several minutes. Used for intraspinal analgesia. See Chapter 5
Transdermal Fentanyl (Duragesic®)	25 µg/hr TD 8–22 mg morphine per day	72		Available in 25-, 50-, 75-, or 100-µg transdermal dosages. Not useful for patients with opioid tolerance or high dosage requirements. If the patch is removed and another analgesic prescribed, begin with half the equinalgesic dose of the new opioid approximately 12–18 hours after removal; the subcutaneous tissue serves as a reservoir and drug continues to be	Primary indication: chronic pain management in patients who are not opioid-naive. Not recommended for acute or postoperative pain management. This noninvasive approach minimizes patient responsibility by delivering drug continuously for up to 72 hours. Some patients have found that the patch needs to be changed before the 72 hours have elapsed

Table continued on following page

TABLE 4-5 *Selected Opioid Analgesics (Continued)*

Generic Name	Equianalgesic Dose (Standard of comparison 10 mg IM morphine)	Approximate Half-Life (hours)	Dosing Interval (hours)	Comments	Clinical Considerations
				available to the patient for up to 18 hours after the patch is removed	Maximum analgesic effect is best evaluated 24 hours after application. Patients may require supplemental short-acting analgesics during this time Fever and external heat sources such as heating pads or electric blankets and hot tubs may increase drug delivery Monitor the patient for analgesic side effects

administered as 0.5-ml boluses every minute (American Pain Society, 1992). The total dose should be titrated to the patient's respiratory rate. The use of antagonists can immediately reverse all opioid effects and result in acute withdrawal that may be complicated by excruciating pain and seizure (AHCPR, 1994).

KEY POINT

When naloxone is needed to reverse opioid-induced respiratory depression, it should be given in incremental doses that help respiratory function, but do not reverse analgesia.

---

10. Patients on chronic opioid therapy generally require a bowel regimen. Tolerance to the constipating effects of opioids does not occur.

11. When it is appropriate to taper the opioid dosage, decrease it slowly. Chronic exposure does produce physical dependence and sudden cessation of an opioid will produce signs and symptoms of withdrawal-agitation, tremors, insomnia, fear, autonomic nervous system hyperexcitability, and increased pain.

12. Use the most appropriate route for the patient's circumstances. Choose the least invasive, most effective, least expensive, and most practical opioid inasmuch as is possible. See Table 4–6. Patients who require chronic opioid dosing and who are on multiple drugs may benefit from a longer-acting preparation that requires fewer scheduled doses. Patients who cannot swallow tablets or capsules may use an elixir, sublingual tablets, or a transdermal preparation. When pain is severe, choose a route with a rapid onset of action. Opioids delivered parenterally work more quickly than oral preparations.

Text continued on page 69

TABLE 4-6 *Opioid Route/Method of Administration*

Route	Indications	Assessment/Monitoring	Comments/Clinical Management	Patient/Family Education
Intravenous	Initial management of moderate to severe pain requiring rapid onset of action. Inability to swallow or tolerate another nonparenteral route. Pain out of control or rapidly escalating Continuous infusion for patients who experience bolus effects such as sedation and rapid return of pain after IV or IM injection	*Peripheral access:* signs/symptoms of infection, infiltration, or inflammation at site *Central access:* signs/symptoms of infection, infiltration, or inflammation; catheter dislodgment or patency	When high dosages are required, sedative toxicity from opioid preservatives may be obviated by preservative-free solution Continuous infusion should be preceded by a period of repetitive IV bolusing with the same drug to determine drug requirements and continuous dosage	*Peripheral access:* signs/symptoms of infiltration, inflammation, and infection; procedure for handling infiltration *Central access:* site care (dressing changes); catheter care
Intramuscular	Short-term use of medications in circumstances where an intravenous route is impossible or impractical	Tissue inflammation and breakdown Excessive bleeding	Not recommended for chronic use—administration is painful Peak effect at 30-60 minutes	Rotation of sites Adequacy of muscle mass Administration techniques

Route	Indications	Contraindications/Assessment	Considerations	Patient/Family Teaching
			Duration of action decreases rapidly compared to the oral route Contraindicated in thrombocytopenic patients Clarify orders if IM route is the primary one and/or to be used on a long-term basis	
Subcutaneous	IV access impractical or impossible Continued and/or bolus dosing outside the hospital Oral access intolerable: GI obstruction, malabsorption, nausea and vomiting, or inability to swallow	Inflammation, infection, or hard, reddened areas at the site	Avoids presystemic hepatic extraction Skin prep similar to IV placement Can use standard 25- or 27-gauge butterfly needles or adhesive dome type 90° angle 27 g SQ needle Needle site change every 7 days or less with commonly used sites: abdomen, subclavicular area, thighs, and upper arms Rotate needle sites using a body chart	Subcutaneous access device/infusion pump handling Site monitoring Needle changes Drug, side effects, complications Steps to take if analgesia inadequate or excessive sedation occurs in the home setting

Table continued on following page

TABLE 4-6 *Opioid Route/Method of Administration (Continued)*

ROUTE	INDICATIONS	ASSESSMENT/MONITORING	COMMENTS/CLINICAL MANAGEMENT	PATIENT/FAMILY EDUCATION
			Chemical irritation and hardened areas at the site may be managed with frequent site changes and/or decrease in infusate concentration Transparent dressing to secure access If infection occurs, change site access and use hot packs and topical ointment	
Oral	Route of choice for those with an intact GI tract	Ability to swallow Functioning of GI tract Nausea/vomiting	Slower onset and long duration of action If sustained release preparation is ordered, confirm that the schedule corresponds with duration of action (8–12 hours)	Necessity for taking "pills" on scheduled basis or as ordered Notify physician if patient is unable to tolerate this route
Sublingual/buccal	Inability to swallow GI tract compromised, but oral management remains viable	Integrity of sublingual, buccal mucosa	Bypasses hepatic extraction by direct absorption into the capillary bed	Proper placement of tablet

		Equianalgesic estimates vary based on absorption, bioavailability, and serum drug levels. Estimates anecdotally seem more closely allied with the parenteral rather than the oral route. Careful dosage titration with individual patients is recommended	
		Buccal route may be preferred over the sublingual as the latter promotes salivation and swallowing, which diminishes potency of the opioid	
		Unpalatable taste may occur with buccal administration	
Rectal	Oral route contraindicated Moderate opioid dosage requirements	Partially avoids hepatic first-pass metabolism as rectal venous drainage occurs via the portal and peripheral venous circulations	Proper insertion of suppository
	Integrity of rectal mucosa Platelet and white count levels adequate		

Table continued on following page

TABLE 4-6 *Opioid Route/Method of Administration* (Continued)

ROUTE	INDICATIONS	ASSESSMENT/MONITORING	COMMENTS/CLINICAL MANAGEMENT	PATIENT/FAMILY EDUCATION
			Dosage titration based on patient response	
			Contraindicated if the patients is neutropenic or thrombocytopenic	
			Use generous amounts of lubricant to minimize discomfort	
			Hydromorphone, oxymorphone, and morphine available in rectal preparations	
Transdermal	Mild to moderate pain requiring continuous administration	Skin integrity	Avoids hepatic first-pass metabolism	Replacement schedule
	Oral route impractical or impossible	Fever (increases absorption)	Dosage equianalgesia is based on manufacturer's recommendation and should be titrated carefully	Application of patch
			Replace every 72 hours or less as necessary	
			See Fentanyl (Duragesic®) on opioid analgesic chart	

ATYPICAL ANALGESICS

Atypical analgesics are nonopioid preparations used primarily in the treatment of other conditions and not typically associated with pain management. They may potentiate the analgesic effects of the opioids, act as analgesics themselves, or be used to treat associated symptoms that exacerbate the pain. They are commonly referred to as *adjuvant analgesics* in the sense that nonopioid and opioid analgesics serve as the primary agent, whereas the atypical analgesic functions as a coanalgesic. These agents include anticonvulsants; local anesthetics and antiarryhthmics; antidepressants; and corticosteroids. Anticonvulsants, local anesthetics and antiarryhthmics, and antidepressants are primarily used to treat neuropathic pain syndromes. Corticosteroids may be used to relieve painful syndromes associated with malignant disease, inflammation, or edema.

Anticonvulsants as well as local anesthetics block ion channels, preventing the generation of the action potential (pain signal) along the neuronal path. Anticonvulsants seem to be particularly effective in suppressing the sharp, "shooting" feature of pain. Phenytoin (Dilantin®) has demonstrated efficacy in the treatment of trigeminal neuralgia, poststroke pain, and diabetic neuropathy. Carbamazepine (Tegretol®) is superior to phenytoin in treating trigeminal neuralgia and has also been used successfully in the treatment of diabetic neuropathy, postherpetic neuralgia, and postsympathectomy pain.

Local anesthetics have been used for some time by anesthesiologists to block nerve conduction for surgical anesthesia and to provide analgesia to manage acute pain. They are used in tandem with epidural opioids to manage obstetrical pain, postoperative pain, and cancer pain. They are injected into painful areas to relieve various musculoskeletal pain syndromes and administered intravenously to treat various types of neuropathic pain as well as migraine headaches. Currently their role in the management of chronic pain is increasing because of the "rejuvenation" of systemic administration.

Many surveys report that local anesthetics are effective for radiculopathies, arachnoiditis, trigeminal neuralgia, phantom pain, postherpetic neuralgia, and diabetic polyneuropathy. The local anesthetics used in these surveys included lidocaine (LidoPen®), the recommended agent for IV therapy; procaine (Novacain®); chloroprocaine (Nesacaine®); and tocainide (Tonocard®). In one randomized trial a group of patients obtained pain relief from lidocaine and maintained it with mexiletine (Mexitil®), an oral antiarrhythmic. Antiarrhythmics suppress spontaneous neuronal firing by blocking ion channels or block alpha-adrenergic stimulation of nerve fibers, thus interfering with the transmission of the pain signal.

Duration of effect is partially determined by the local anesthetic's protein-binding capability. For example, procaine may provide 30 minutes of relief when used for a brachial plexus blockade whereas bupivicaine (Marcaine®) will provide relief for up to 10 hours. Although they can be temporarily effective, the disadvantage of using a local anesthetic procedurally for chronic pain (e.g., epidural injection of corticosteroid and Marcaine® for low-back pain) is its time-limited efficacy. Systemic administration on a chronic basis has demonstrated extended analgesic relief. A successful monitored trial with an intravenous local anesthetic such as lidocaine should generally precede the use of oral agents (e.g., mexilitene and tocainide) on an outpatient basis. Dosages used for pain are in the ranges recommended for control of cardiac arrhythmias. Side effects include tinnitus, paresthesias, tremor, dizziness, and nausea.

Antidepressant medications are hypothesized to be effective in relieving neuropathies because of their inhibitory activity of synaptic norepinephrine and/or serotonin reuptake. Clinical experience with selective serotonergic agents (e.g., fluoxetine [Prozac®] for chronic pain relief has been disappointing, which could mean that a primary serotonergic mechanism is unlikely. Antidepressant agents that are primarily noradrenergic (e.g., nortriptyline [Pamelor®]) and those that inhibit norepinephrine and serotonin (e.g., amitryptyline [Elavil®]) have demonstrated more efficacy. Therapeutic advantages include (1) significant relief unattainable by any other analgesic or nonanalgesic agent; (2) early onset of analgesia; (3) efficacy with low doses and serum levels; and (4) analgesia independent of antidepressant effect.

Antidepressant medications are well absorbed from the GI tract and have long half-lives (e.g., 20 hours for amitriptyline). They may be administered in a single daily dose given at bedtime that may decrease side effects and allow the sedative effects to aid in sleep. They do have significant side effect profiles. Dry mouth and constipation, very common with amitriptyline and imipramine (Tofranil®), are less common with nortriptyline and desipramine (Norpramin®). For most patients, dry mouth, a common anticholinergic effect, comes in tandem with pain relief and can be managed with lozenges and/or methylcellulose mouth sprays. Constipation is generally controlled with diet and stool softeners. Patients should be informed about the possibilities of postural hypotension, tachycardia, impotence, priapism, urinary retention, blurred vision, confusion, hallucinations, and excessive drowsiness, side effects most likely to lead to discontinuation of therapy.

It is reasonable to trial antidepressant therapy if there are no contraindications, for these agents may be the only source of relief. Although it is clear that not all antidepressants are efficacious and a percentage of patients receive no or at best inadequate relief, a trial period is the only definitive answer. Antidepressant agents have been most successfully used in the treatment of postherpetic neuralgia and painful diabetic neuropathy, conditions characterized by dull aching or burning pain. The dose-producing analgesia is variable and starting doses are recommended to be in the low to moderate range with subsequent increases made dependent on the clinical response.

Corticosteroids may have direct analgesic effects as well as add to the analgesic effect of opioids. They are hormones that have been demonstrated to inhibit prostaglandin synthesis, reduce capillary permeability and peritumoral edema, and reduce spontaneous discharge in injured nerves. They have been used systemically to treat acute nerve compression, increased intracranial pressure, lymphedema, spinal cord compression, superior vena cava syndrome, and to treat pain secondary to bone metastases. Epidural

Text continued on page 76

TABLE 4-7 *Selected Atypical Analgesics*

ANALGESIC	INDICATIONS	EFFECTS	SIDE EFFECTS	COMMENTS
Tricyclic antidepressants Amitriptyline (Elavil®) Desipramine (Norpramin®) Imipramine (Tofranil®) Nortriptyline (Pamelor®)	Neuropathic pain: post-herpetic neuralgia and diabetic neuropathy Cancer pain complicated by depression or insomnia Migraine headaches Fibromyalgia	Improves mood Relieves depression Promotes sleep when taken at bedtime Direct analgesic effect Augments analgesic response to opioids	Dry mouth Urinary retention Blurred vision Constipation Sleepiness Light-headedness Postural hypotension	Begin with moderate dosage and titrate up; analgesic dose less than antidepressant dose Needs adequate trial period (2 weeks or more) to reach steady serum state and determine analgesic efficacy Administer at bedtime due to potential for sleepiness, lightheadedness, and mild hypotension Must distinguish between side effects that are tolerable and treatable and those that are severe and unbearable *Amitriptyline* has most supportive clinical data and is least costly; may have dose-limiting sedative and anticholinergic effects *Nortriptyline* and *desipramine* are markedly less sedating with less anticholinergic effect

Agents	Indications	Mechanism of Action	Side Effects	Nursing Considerations
				Dry mouth seems to accompany pain relief
				Preexistence of glaucoma is a concern but not a contraindication; tricyclics can be used if pilocarpine eye drops are used; best choice is *desipramine*
				Avoid use following a myocardial infarction
Anticonvulsants Phenytoin (Dilantin®) Carbamazepine (Tegretol®) Clonazepam (Klonopin®) Gabapentin (Neurontin®)	Neuropathic pain secondary to surgical trauma Postherpetic neuralgia Diabetic neuropathy Trigeminal neuralgia Poststroke pain	Suppresses spontaneous neuronal firing by blocking ion channels May increase concentration of GABA (inhibitory neurotransmitter) in CNS	Gingival hyperplasia (Dilantin®) Neutropenia and hepatic dysfunction (Tegretol®) Nystagmus Ataxia/slurred speech/mental confusion GI effects	Assess serum levels for therapeutic efficacy; analgesic levels similar to anticonvulsant levels Assess for sequelae: Tegretol® requires liver function tests and neutrophil counts Administer with food to minimize GI irritation Monitor pharmacokinetics: dramatically influenced by calcium channel blockers and some antibiotics and anticoagulants; known to decrease effect of steroids

Table continued on following page

TABLE 4-7 *Selected Atypical Analgesics (Continued)*

Analgesic	Indications	Effects	Side Effects	Comments
Corticosteroids Dexamethasone (Decadron®) Prednisone (Deltasone®) Methylprednisolone (Medrol®, Solu-Medrol®) Cortisone Acetate Hydrocortisone (Cortef®, Solu-Cortef®)	Bone metastases Lymphedema Brachial or lumbosacral plexopathy Spinal cord compression Superior vena cava syndrome Acute nerve compression Increased intracranial pressure Epidural injections for pain secondary to herniated disc, spinal stenosis, laminectomy, and neck problems	Anti-inflammatory activity Decreases edema Increases appetite (time limited) Elevates mood in nondepressed individuals	Immediate Hypertension Hyperglycemia Immunosuppression Mood disorders Restlessness/agitation/insomnia Fluid retention Gastric irritation Gastric ulceration (when used in combination with NSAIDs) Long-term: osteoporosis	May be administered IV, IM, SQ, PO; and topically Contraindicated in presence of active bleeding or systemic infections *Cortisone* and *prednisone* require activation in the liver and may not be effective in the presence of hepatic dysfunction *Hydrocortisone, prednisone,* and *prednisolone* need to be administered more frequently than *dexamethasone* High doses are used on a short-term basis for patients with severe pain secondary to bony involvement or compression of neural structures Low doses may be used for extended periods when benefits of therapy are greater than risks Optimal drug and dosing regimens not established

Local anesthetics/antiarrhythmics				
Lidocaine (LidoPen®, Xylocaine®)	Postherpetic neuralgia	Suppresses spontaneous neuronal firing by blocking ion channels	Heartburn	Systemic administration (IV, SQ, oral) can provide relief for some types of chronic pain
Procaine (Novacain®)	Diabetic neuropathy	May block alpha adrenergic stimulation of nerve fibers	Nausea	A trial of IV lidocaine is desirable to determine analgesic efficacy preceding the use of oral mexilitene
Bupivicaine (Marcaine®)	Poststroke pain		Unsteady gait	Lower doses used for pain relief
Mexilitene (Mexitil®) [oral]	Dermal analgesia prior to intravenous catheter placement, venipuncture, and split skin graft harvest		Cardiac effects	Administer oral agents with food to minimize GI effects
Tocainide (Tonocard®) [oral]			Paresthesias, tremor, dizziness	EMLA® must be applied to intact skin under an occlusive dressing for at least 1 hour before IV catheter placement and venipuncture and 2 hours before split skin graft harvesting
Lidocaine/prilocaine (EMLA®) [topical emulsion]				

injections have provided relief for radiculopathy from herniated discs and spinal stenosis, laminectomy, and neck problems.

They are well absorbed orally but can also be administered intravenously, intramuscularly, subcutaneously, and topically. They have both immediate and long-term toxic profiles that require monitoring (Table 4–7). Although corticosteroids have been demonstrated to be helpful in varied clinical situations, the relief they provide seems to be time-limited, and the benefit temporary. The ideal dosage and schedule have not been determined and require further study.

Neuroleptics, which are generally used to treat psychoses and other psychiatric disorders, also are used as adjunctive analgesics. The best known, methotrimeprazine (Levoprome®), is a phenothiazine that seems to provide analgesia through α-adrenergic stimulation. It can be helpful for patients who are opioid tolerant or who have dose-limiting opioid side effects.

Given the complex nature of the pain experience, it is expected that adjuvant analgesic preparations may be added to the pharmacotherapeutic regimen. In addition to those preparations already mentioned that seem to have primary analgesic effect, medications are used that treat multiple problems secondary to the illness and analgesic treatment experience. Common *antiemetics* include Vistaril®, Compazine®, Torecan®, and Reglan®. Up to 40% of patients receiving opioids develop mild to moderate nausea. This side effect generally decreases after 2 to 3 days of repeated opioid dosing. Pain exacerbates and is exacerbated by anxiety. For selected patients it may be appropriate to include an *anxiolytic* in the therapeutic regimen. Ativan® and Xanax® are common choices. Insomnia may compound the difficulties of the pain experience. Lack of sleep imposes further burdens by depleting the individual's finite physiologic and psychologic resources. A sleeping aid may be added to the therapeutic regimen with consideration given to half-life as well as concomitant medications with CNS effects.

The complexities of the pain experience cannot be reduced to a single treatment approach, but there is no doubt that analgesic therapy is the major contributor to the relief of acute, chronic nonmalignant, and chronic malignant pain. The nonopioid and opioid analgesics are used concurrently or alone to treat a multitude of acute painful syndromes. Chronic pain management, although employing a multimodal approach that focuses on nonpharmacologic interventions, nevertheless incorporates nonopioids, opioid, and atypical preparations for pain relief over time, possibly over the lifetime. Because every medication carries its own side effect profile, it is imperative that clinicians involved in the treatment of pain understand the risks and benefits of each therapy.

BIBLIOGRAPHY

American Pain Society. (1992). *Principles of analgesic use in the treatment of acute pain and chronic cancer pain* (3rd ed.). Skokie, IL: American Pain Society.

Backonja, M. (1994). Local anesthetics as adjuvant analgesics. *Journal of Pain and Symptom Management 9*(8), 491–499.

Beaver, W.T. (1990). Nonsteroidal anti-inflammatory analgesics in cancer pain. In K.M. Foley et al. (Eds.), *Advances in pain research and theory* (Vol. 16, pp. 109–131). New York: Raven.

Benedetti, C., & Butler, S.H. (1990). Systemic analgesics. In J.J. Bonica (Ed.), *The management of pain* (2nd ed., pp. 1640–1676). Philadelphia: Lea & Febiger.

Cherney, N.I., Thaler, H.T., Friedlander-Klar, H., Lapin, J., Foley, K.M., Houde, R., & Portenoy, R.K. (1994). Opioid responsiveness of cancer pain syndromes caused by neuropathic or nociceptive mechanisms: A combined analysis of controlled, single-dose studies. *Neurology 44,* 857–861.

DeBoer, A.G., De Leede, L.G.J., & Breimer, D.D. (1984). Drug absorption by sublingual and rectal routes. *British Journal of Anesthesiology, 56,* 69–82.

DeStoutz, N.D., Bruera, E., & Suarez-Almazor, M. (1995). Opioid rotation for toxicity reduction in terminal cancer patients. *Journal of Pain and Symptom Management 10*(5), 378–384.

Fromm, G.H. (1994). Baclofen as an adjuvant analgesic. *Journal of Pain and Symptom Management 9*(8), 500–509.

Galer, B.S., Coyle, N., Pasternak, G.W., & Portenoy, R.K. (1992). Individual variability in the response to different opioids: Report of five cases. *Pain 49,* 87–91.

Hagen, N.A., Foley, K.M., Cerbone, D.J., Portenoy, R.K., & Inturrisi, C.E. (1991). Chronic nausea and morphine-6-glucuronide. *Journal of Pain and Symptom Management 6* (3), 125–128.

Jacox, A., Carr, D.B., and Payne, R., et al. (1994). *Management of cancer pain. Clinical practice guideline.* (AHCPR Publication No. 94-0592). Rockville, MD: Agency for Health Care Policy and Research, U.S. Department of Health and Human Services.

Joel, G., Hardman, J.G., Limbard, E.L., Molinoff, P.B., Ruddon, R.W., & Gilman, A.G. (Eds.). (1996). *Goodman and Gilman's the pharmacological basis of therapeutics.* New York: McGraw-Hill.

Kaiko, R.F., Foley, K.M., Grabinski, P.Y., et al. (1983). Central nervous system excitatory effects of meperidine in cancer patients. *Annals of Neurology 13*, 180–185.

Lehmann, K.A., & Zech, Detlev. (1992). Transdermal fentanyl: Clinical pharmacology. *Journal of Pain and Symptom Management 7*(3S), S8–S17.

Miller, D.R. (1981). Combination use of non-steroidal anti-inflammatory drugs. *Drug Intelligence and Clinical Pharmacy 15*, 3–7.

Monks, R. (1990). Psychotropic drugs. In J.J. Bonica (Ed.), *The management of pain* (2nd ed., pp. 1676–1690). Philadelphia: Lea & Febiger.

Portenoy, R.K., & Hagen, N.R. (1990). Breakthrough pain: Definition, characteristics, and prevalence. *Pain 41*, 273–282.

Portenoy, R.K., Foley, K.M., & Inturrisi, C.E. (1990). The nature of opioid responsiveness and its implications for neuropathic pain: New hypotheses derived from studies of opioid infusions. *Pain 43*, 273–286.

Reddy, S., & Patt, R.B. (1994). The benzodiazepines as adjuvant analgesics. *Journal of Pain and Symptom Management 9*, 510–514.

Sindrup, S.H., Arendt-Nielse, L., Brosen, K., et al. (1992). The effects of quinidine on the analgesic effect of codeine. *European Journal of Clinical Pharmacology 42*, 587–591.

Watanabe, S., & Bruera, E. (1994). Corticosteroids as adjuvant analgesics. *Journal of Pain and Symptom Management 9*(7), 442–445.

Watson, C.P.N. (1994). Antidepressant drugs as adjuvant analgesics. *Journal of Pain and Symptom Management 9*(6), 392–405.

5
Alternate Administration of Opioids

PATIENT-CONTROLLED ANALGESIA

Patient-controlled analgesia (PCA) is a drug-delivery approach that employs an external infusion pump to deliver opioids on a "patient demand," or bolus basis. The patient-controlled dosing is driven by the patient's need for analgesia, and the pump's preprogrammed instructions to deliver on demand an identified dosage of opioid at specified intervals. The program cannot be overridden by the patient. In addition to the patient-initiated bolus dose, most pumps also have the capacity to deliver a continuous infusion, which may be used in combination with patient-initiated doses. The continuous infusion is designed to provide a strategized proportion of the patient's total pain relief with the remainder of the analgesic need covered by the patient initiated bolus doses. The proportions of total pain relief assigned to the continuous infusion and bolus dosing capacity depend on the nature and extent of the pain and patient circumstances.

Past experience with PCA has documented (1) improved pain relief with minimal sedation and less overall dosage; (2) more finely tuned drug titration with lower potential for overdosage; (3) decreased delay between request for analgesia and relief; (4) decreased dependency on nursing staff; (5) earlier mobilization with increased pulmonary toilet; and (6) decreased patient anxiety resulting from inadequate or poorly managed pain relief.

Patients are selected based on their need for repeated parenteral dosing for moderate to severe pain, their ability to understand and follow instructions, and their willingness to employ this method. Those who are unable to understand the instructions or who have physical disabilities that preclude the actual manipulation of the pump would be poor candidates for this type of analgesic delivery. There is some controversy about using this method for patients with a prior history of substance abuse. The issue does not center on the patient's need for pain relief, but rather on the patient and/or health care provider's reluctance to give the patient some control over the analgesic intake.

Patient-controlled analgesia can be delivered through a variety of routes. Although it was initially developed for use intravenously, subcutaneous and epidural administration are increasingly more commonplace. As we learn to manage pain more effectively and deliver that management in a variety of settings across the illness continuum, alternative routes are not only practical but necessary.

Inpatient Usage

Postoperative Analgesia/Trauma

Historically, PCA was developed to manage pain more effectively in the postoperative setting. The practicality and effectiveness of this analgesic-delivery method have extended its use to other patient populations. Moderate to severe burn and trauma pain responds well to this management approach. Conventional "as-needed" intramuscular dosing, a common analgesic approach for postoperative and trauma patients, has two primary disadvantages. Pain relief is delayed in the multistep process of patient recognition of pain and request for analgesia, the clinician's preparation and administration of the analgesic, and the analgesic's onset of action. As-needed dosing adequate to provide relief for 3 to 4 hours at a time produces large swings in serum analgesic levels that can result in over- and undermedication.

Severe pain that decreases in intensity as tissue heals lends itself to this dosing method. On-demand dosing alone or in combination with continuous infusion may be used for analgesic relief. The patient-initiated dose, usually moderate in nature, is preprogrammed to be delivered on demand at short intervals (e.g., every 10–15 minutes).

In the acute care setting PCA is usually administered via an intravenous route. Indwelling intravenous access, common in multiple patient populations, provides a route with a rapid onset of action and precludes the further discomfort of an intramuscular injection. Analgesics commonly used include morphine, hydromorphone (Dilaudid®), and meperidine (Demerol®).

Analgesia for Chronic/Incident Pain

Other inpatient populations may be well served by the use of PCA. The on-demand bolus capacity of PCA allows rapid titration and determination of the overall analgesic dosage required in a 24-hour period. Chronic cancer pain with episodes of incident, or breakthrough, pain that has not responded well to less invasive routes or that is severe in nature and rapidly escalating can be effectively managed using this method. Management includes a combination of continuous and PCA dosing. The cumulative 24-hour dosage needed for adequate relief would then serve as the baseline dose for the following 24 hours. Under these circumstances, the intravenous route with its rapid onset of action is the most efficient and effective way to control the pain and titrate the dosage. Once the patient is maintained on a stable dose and being readied for discharge from the acute care setting, alternatives include: (1) converting the parenteral dose to an equianalgesic oral dose; (2) establishing stable intravenous access for patients requiring significant doses of opioids and discharging them with an intravenous ambulatory PCA device; or (3) converting the intravenous route to a subcutaneous one. The last choice depends on overall dosage required and concentration of the drug to be delivered.

Outpatient Usage

Although permanent or long-term indwelling intravenous access devices would support the intravenous route for home care use, subcutaneous administration of analgesics is more practical in the home care setting and is the route of choice for those without dependable venous access. Reliability and ease of access by a trained layperson make it sensible and dependable. The subcutaneous tissue contains a dense capillary network that absorbs the opioid solution. Blood levels rise gradually, but ultimately equal those obtained from an intravenous infusion.

This route may be used for patient populations for whom intravenous access is not possible or practical, for those with significant chronic and breakthrough pain requiring continuous infusions and on-demand doses of opioid, and for those unable to tolerate the oral route because of decreased consciousness, GI obstruction, malabsorption, and/or uncontrollable nausea and vomiting.

Both morphine and hydromorphone come in concentrated formulations that allow significant doses to be delivered in relatively small volumes, an important consideration for subcutaneous absorption. Patients and family members can be taught to change sites and manage the ambulatory infusion pump, which obviates the need for an emergency visit by a trained health care professional if the current site is no longer suitable.

CASE STUDY

Adele is a 35-year-old female, posthysterectomy. She weighs 170 pounds, is 5'11" tall, and is a marathon runner. She is admitted to the surgical unit from the recovery room. During her stay in the recovery room she received 25 mg Demerol® intravenously 3 times, the last dose having been given 45 minutes ago. She immediately reports to her admitting nurse that her pain is "out of control." Upon further questioning, she rates her pain to be a 10 on a scale of 0 to 10. The clinician contacts her physician who orders a PCA pump with morphine at 2 mg/hour and a 2-mg bolus dose that may be accessed every 15 minutes. He further orders a loading dose of morphine at 2 mg every 5 minutes up to 14 mg until Adele reports comfort or becomes drowsy. Adele receives 14 mg of morphine as a loading dose and reports her pain to be reduced to 4 on a scale of 0 to 10. The PCA pump is initiated, and she uses two 2-mg bolus doses every hour from 12 noon until 8:30 P.M. She reports that she can keep her pain under control only if she gives herself those extra doses every hour. The clinician again contacts her physician and reports that Adele is averaging 6 mg of morphine/hour. Her respiratory rate is 16, her pulse 100, and her blood pressure 128/86. The continuous infusion of morphine is increased to 4 mg/hour for the next 10 hours with the bolus dose to remain as previously ordered. She requires two bolus doses per hour for the next 2 hours and then is able to sleep comfortably through the night as long as she does not have to move excessively.

On the second postoperative day she tolerates oral intake and is started on an NSAID four times a day. The continuous opioid infusion is discontinued with the bolus dose capacity remaining intact. As her bolus needs diminish, she is converted to an oral opioid on an as-needed basis and discharged the third postoperative day.

SPINAL ANALGESIA

The discovery of opioid receptors in the spinal column prompted initial clinical work in the administration of opioids at the spinal level. The efficacy of this method is due to the interaction between the opioid and opioid receptor complexes in the dorsal horn of the spinal cord and has proven effective in treating certain acute and chronic pain conditions. Subsequently, local anesthetics (e.g., bupivacaine [Marcaine®]) and clonidine, an α_2-adrenoreceptor agonist, have been added to spinal analgesic regimens. Their analgesic mechanisms of action differ markedly from that of the opioids, and they are frequently used in combination with the opioids to maximize analgesic relief. In some instances, such as during the acute postoperative period or in the initial treatment of chronic malignant pain, opioids may be used as single agents. The pharmacologic section of this chapter provides details on their use.

Epidural analgesia is used postoperatively for multiple types of surgery and employs a temporary catheter. Postoperative epidural analgesia has proven to be very effective and promotes good pulmonary toilet and early ambulation. Patients with intractable pain also are candidates for spinal analgesia. A successful trial with opioids and/or local anesthetic via a temporary catheter commonly precedes the placement of a permanent epidural or intrathecal catheter. There are fewer side effects with epidural and **intrathecal** analgesia than with systemically administered opioids because of the relatively low drug dosages required for spinal delivery compared to the much higher dosages used systemically. Because epidural and intrathecal analgesia are invasive therapies, not without risk, and require standardized and responsible postplacement care, they should be used for chronic pain management only when maximal doses of opioids and adjuvant analgesics administered through other routes have failed to provide adequate relief.

Intrathecal Therapy

Intrathecal therapy is traditionally reserved for chronic pain states. The catheter tip is placed in the subarachnoid space between the dura mater and the spinal cord (Figure 5–1). This placement allows the drug to diffuse immediately into the cerebrospinal fluid and then into the spinal cord, where it binds with opioid receptors. Although a small amount of drug may be absorbed into surrounding blood vessels, the close proximity of the drug to the opioid receptors produces analgesia with the least amount of drug in comparison to all other routes. Catheter tip placement directly into the subarachnoid space requires an administrative system that maximally protects the patient from infection. A "closed" system is typically used, which is comprised of the intrathecally placed catheter subcutaneously tunneled and connected to a surgically implanted pump in the abdomen. The pump may be percutaneously programmed via a computer to deliver the required analgesic doses and is accessed percutaneously for reservoir refills.

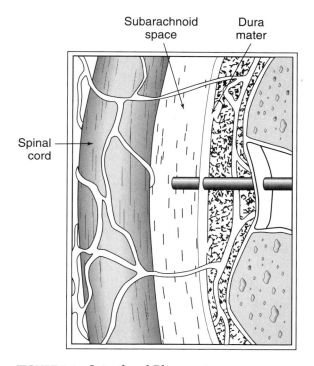

FIGURE 5–1   *Intrathecal Placement*
The catheter tip is located in the subarachnoid space between the dura mater and the spinal cord.

Intrathecal therapy selection criteria for cancer patients include (1) inadequate pain relief despite escalating doses delivered per conventional routes; (2) intolerable/unmanageable side effects from systemic opioids; and (3) life expectancy greater than 3 months. Patient selection criteria for those with nonmalignant pain are less straightforward and more controversial. Suggested selection criteria include (1) therapy of last resort; (2) baseline neurologic exam; and (3) psychometric testing and psychologic evaluation documenting that pain is not primarily of psychologic origin. A positive response to a trial of epidural or intrathecal infusion therapy should be documented before the permanent catheter is placed.

Epidural Therapy

The epidural route is more commonplace and is used for both acute and chronic pain management. The catheter tip is located in the space between the spinal vertebrae and the dura mater, the outer protective covering of the spinal cord and spinal fluid (Figure 5–2). The epidural space consists of spinal nerve extensions, fat, and an extensive web of thin-walled veins. The opioid diffuses from the epidural space across the dura mater into the cerebrospinal fluid and subsequently into the spinal cord where it binds with the opioid receptors. Complicating factors include (1) a thick dura mater that may limit drug diffusion into the cerebrospinal fluid; (2) drug uptake into the general

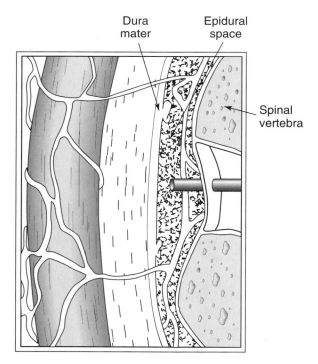

Dura mater   Epidural space

Spinal vertebra

FIGURE 5–2   *Epidural Placement*
The catheter tip is located between the spinal vertebrae and the dura mater.

circulation and the cerebral venous system via the vast blood supply in the epidural space; and (3) saturation of opioid receptors resulting in higher cerebrospinal fluid and blood levels, but no corresponding increase in pain relief.

Indications for epidural therapy include, but are not limited to, (1) short-term relief via a temporary catheter for thoracic, abdominal, or orthopedic surgical patients; (2) multiple trauma pain; (3) acute pain conditions, where mobility and full lung expansion in the immediate postoperative period are especially important; and (4) chronic cancer pain that does not respond to conventional aggressive opioid intervention or that has required opioid therapy that produces intolerable and unmanageable side effects. Epidural analgesia may be produced by intermittent injections, continuous infusions, or a combination of the two. Patient-controlled epidural analgesia, which allows the patient the ability to administer bolus doses for **breakthrough pain** via an ambulatory pump is becoming more commonplace as patients are increasingly being cared for at home as they near the end of the disease continuum.

For selected surgical populations where surgical pain is expected to be of relatively short duration, a single epidural injection of morphine may be adequate. Other surgical patient populations may require intermittent injections or a low-dose continuous infusion. Morphine, sufentanil, fentanyl, and/or bupivacaine are typically used, and current research is examining the efficacy of clonidine for postoperative pain. Some clinicians argue that a combination of opioid/local anesthetic produces superior analgesia to an opioid alone during mobilization and coughing. Whatever the analgesic regimen ultimately proves to be, benefits of effective epidural analgesia include improved respiratory function, earlier mobilization and return of bowel function, heightened alertness, and a feeling of well-being. At the same time there are identified risks to epidural therapy. Respiratory depression is most commonly identified, but hypotension, migration of the epidural catheter into the subarachnoid space, epidural abscess formation, and epidural hematoma are infrequent, but to be taken seriously.

Chronic malignant pain is typically treated with a continuous infusion of opioid and/or local anesthetic with or without bolus doses for breakthrough pain. Intractable chronic malignant pain that does not respond to opioid/local anesthetic therapy may be treated with clonidine. Successful analgesia with clonidine is more common in those cancer patients with neuropathic pain. Cancer patients who are managed with epidural analgesia have been shown to require less analgesia, to be more alert, and less depressed, and to have an increased ability to resume daily activities within the constraints of their disease state.

Pharmacologic Considerations

Varied pharmacologic agents are used to provide spinal analgesia. Opioids such as morphine, hydromorphone (Dilaudid®), fentanyl, and sufentanil are used singly or in combination with bupivacaine (Marcaine®), a local anesthetic. The high concentration of opioid receptors in the dorsal horn of the spinal cord renders opioid analgesics particularly effective at reduced doses. This altered dosage decreases the incidence of central nervous system (CNS) side effects because of the limited amount of opioid that ascends to the higher brain centers via the cerebrospinal fluid or that is absorbed systemically via the blood supply in the epidural space.

Clonidine, an α_2-adrenoreceptor agonist that has traditionally been used as an antihypertensive agent, has been utilized in clinical trials settings to manage intractable cancer pain. As with opioid receptors, there is a high density of adrenoreceptors in the superficial dorsal horn. Activation of the α_2-adrenoreceptors blocks transmission of the ascending pain signal. The high density of those adrenoreceptors makes clonidine an effective analgesic when administered epidurally, but produces poor analgesic results when it is administered systemically:

- Onset and duration of action are determined by solubility and the receptor affinity of the drug.

Lipophilic (lipid-soluble) opioids, such as fentanyl and sufentanil, cross the dura mater rapidly and bind with the opioid receptors, creating segmental analgesia i.e., analgesia limited to a certain area of the body (Figure 5-3). Central nervous system side effects are reduced because the opioid is less inclined to spread rostrally (toward the brain) via the cerebrospinal fluid. Quick diffusion across the dura mater membrane results in a rapid onset and short duration of action. In contrast, hydrophilic (water-soluble) opioids such as morphine and hydromorphone (Dilaudid®) will cross the dura mater more slowly and diffuse widely in the aqueous cerebrospinal fluid. This tendency produces a slower onset of action, greater area of analgesia (more spinal segments covered), and longer duration of analgesia. It also increases the possibility that the opioid will spread rostrally, causing delayed respiratory depression (6–8 hours) and other CNS side effects, such as confusion and sedation.

- Bupivacaine (Marcaine®), a lipophilic local anesthetic, may be used in conjunction with an opioid (Figure 5-3). Local anesthetics produce a nerve blockade that interrupts motor, sensory, and sympathetic function. The extent of the blockade is dependent on the local anesthetic concentration. Use may decrease the amount of opioid required and can be extremely helpful when the pain has a neuropathic component or when there is unstable bone pain.

- Clonidine provides spinal analgesia that is not reversed by naloxone (Narcan®). This therapy seems to be most effective in patients whose pain is primarily neuropathic in origin. Nausea, vomiting, pruritus, and urinary retention are not common side effects (Table 5–1).

- Dosage range varies widely depending on pain intensity and prior opioid experience. Equianalgesic morphine conversion is: oral to intravenous 3:1; intravenous to epidural 3:1. Thus, 90 mg of oral morphine/day = 30 mg of parenteral

TABLE 5–1 *Intraspinal Analgesic Agents*

Solubility: Drug Options	Mechanism of Action	Onset of Action	Receptor Affinity; Duration of Action	Distribution	Side Effects
Hydrophilic: opioid examples: morphine hydromorphone	Binds to opioid receptor sites and inhibits release of substance P	Slow 10–30 min, 15 min	Strong: prolonged 6–24 hr, 10–15 hr	Wide: tends to cover all spinal segments	Higher risk of CNS side effects: mental status changes and respiratory depression
Lipophilic: opioid examples: fentanyl sufentanil	Binds to opioid receptor sites and inhibits release of substance P	Rapid 10–15 min, 5–10 min	Weak: short 2–3 hr 2–4 hr	Narrow: highly segmental analgesia	Lower risk of CNS side effects Less pruritus and nausea than with other opioids
Lipophilic: clonidine	Alpha-2 adrenoreceptor agonist that modulates ascending pain signal Reduces substance P release	Rapid 20 min	Strong Unclear	Narrow: highly segmental analgesia	Decreased blood pressure and heart rate Sedation No major respiratory depressant effects
Lipophilic: bupivacaine (local anesthetic)	Temporarily interrupts transmission of pain impulses at dorsal root ganglion	Rapid 10–30 min	Not applicable: short 4–6 hr	Narrow: highly segmental analgesia	Hypotension, motor weakness and numbness

morphine/day = 10 mg of epidural morphine/day. When converting the patient from systemic opioids to epidural opioids, it may be necessary to titrate the systemic dosage downward while titrating the epidural dosage upward to prevent opioid withdrawal. A 25%–50% decrease per day has been suggested.

- Bupivacaine dosage is typically expressed by the concentration (e.g., 0.15% solution). The dosage ultimately delivered depends on the concentration of the solution, the volume infused, and the side effect profile.

- Pharmacologic agents and solutions injected into the epidural space must be preservative free because of potential neurotoxicity. Preparations containing phenol, formaldehyde, and alcohol have resulted in both CNS and local epidural tissue toxicity.

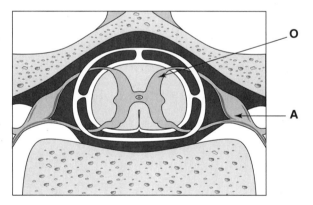

FIGURE 5–3 *Action of Epidural Medications*
The efficacy of opioids and local anesthetics is mediated by their proximity to the site of action. Opioids block pain pathways by binding to receptor sites in the dorsal horn of the spinal cord (O). Local anesthetics interfere with the transmission of the pain signal primarily in the dorsal root ganglion before it enters the spinal cord (A).

TABLE 5–2 *Potential Side Effects of Spinal Analgesia*

Side Effect	Circumstances	Management Principles
Respiratory depression	*Risk Factors:* limited exposure to opioid analgesics, advanced age, significant opioid dosages, concomitant use of other CNS depressants. More likely to occur after large bolus dose vs. continuous infusion *Early:* result of vascular uptake and redistribution *Late:* rostral spread of water soluble opioids affecting respiratory center. Risk greatest during initial therapy	Monitor for signs of drowsiness/sedation. This precedes respiratory depression Intravenous naloxone titrated slowly to effect. Reduce the risk for return of pain and withdrawal by careful titration Short half-life of naloxone may require repeated administration
Extreme drowsiness or sedation	Result of rostral spread of water-soluble opioids affecting respiratory center Associated with high opioid doses or concomitant use of tranquilizers, sedatives, or systemic opioids	Monitor carefully as this precedes respiratory depression If administering bolus doses, hold 1–2 doses. Reduce the dose per physician's orders. If continuous infusion, reduce dose per physician's orders
Gastrointestinal effects	Constipation: common with morphine Nausea/vomiting: results from rostral spread of the opioid to the vomiting center and chemoreceptor trigger zone. Tolerance develops rapidly	Titrate bowel regimen to effect Intravenous antiemetics may be indicated

Urinary retention	May result from decreased parasympathetic flow from spinal cord, rostral spread of the opioid to micturition center in the brain, or direct effect of the opioid on the spinal cord resulting in altered bladder tone Occurs generally in elderly males or persons with pre-existing bladder disorders Usually resolves within 48 hours	Monitor carefully for retention May require intermittent catheterization or indwelling urinary catheter for a time-limited period
Pruritus	Etiology unknown. Not dose related Can occur for duration of analgesia Usually occurs on face and/or palate	Small doses of diluted naloxone or an oral antihistamine may be tried
Hypotension	Local anesthetics can trigger sympathetic blockade and capillary vasodilation: More pronounced in patients who are volume depleted Usually resolves within 48 hours	May need to administer fluids, volume depending on the patient's cardiac status Reduce local anesthetic concentration
Sensory or motor block	Local anesthetics may cause loss of motor function in the lower extremities and an inability to flex the knees or ankles Tingling, numbness, weakness, or loss of sensation	Reduce local anesthetic concentration or volume delivered

Side Effect Management

Although side effects are not uncommon, they are rarely life-threatening. Epidural acute pain management in the opioid-naive patient is more likely to produce side effects than in cancer patients with a prior history of significant systemic dosing. As mentioned, the rostral spread of the water-soluble opioids, such as morphine, to the supraspinal level may cause the same CNS side effects as those seen with systemically administered opioids. The local anesthetic bupivacaine has its own side effect profile that differs from the opioid analgesics. Its blockade of motor, sensory, and sympathetic function can result in hypotension and numbness, and tingling and weakness in the lower extremities. Clonidine's primary side effects are a decrease in blood pressure and heart rate, and sedation. Clonidine has no major respiratory depressant effects (Table 5–2).

Methods of Spinal Drug Delivery

The system chosen for delivering spinal analgesia depends on the nature of the disease and/or therapy, projected duration of therapy, and technical support systems available. A temporary external catheter inserted percutaneously into the epidural space is indicated for short-term pain management. It is inexpensive, easily inserted, and provides access for continuous infusion and bolus dosing of analgesics. The temporary catheters are commonly used to manage acute, postoperative pain and to trial spinal infusions of opioids and/or local anesthetics prior to permanent catheter placement. This catheter is easily dislodged and carries infection risks. A permanent catheter may be placed for long-term access. This catheter is tunneled from the epidural or intrathecal space to the drug-delivery site and can deliver a continuous infusion with or without intermittent bolus dosing of opioid and/or local anesthetic. There is a decreased risk of dislodgment/migration and a lower incidence of infection than with temporary catheters. However, infection remains the primary risk for any spinal drug-delivery system (Table 5–3).

TABLE 5–3   *Spinal Drug-Delivery Systems*

System	Nursing Implications
Tunneled catheter with anterior exit site for continuous infusion and/or bolus dosing into the epidural space	Risk: infection Site and catheter care
Tunneled catheter accessed percutaneously via implanted port for continuous infusion and/or bolus injections into the epidural space	Risks: infection, needle dislodgment Skin irritation from percutaneous access Site and access care
Tunneled catheter connected to implanted pump with indwelling reservoir programmed and accessed percutaneously for intrathecal therapy	Risk: infection Infrequent reservoir refills No patient-controlled bolus dosing Requires programming and pump-maintenance skills

CASE STUDY

Ingrid is a 52-year-old female with extensive bone metastases and tumor compressing her spinal cord in the lumbar region. At presentation she is paraplegic with significant pain in her lower back and radiating down both of her lower extremities. She has a foley catheter and requires manual disimpaction to pass stool. She rates her pain to be an 8 on a scale of 0 to 10. In addition to maximum daily doses of an NSAID and analgesic doses of an antidepressant, she has been requiring increasingly greater doses of parenteral morphine delivered intravenously. She is becoming confused on the 100 mg of morphine per hour but verbalizes that the pain is "excruciating."

A temporary epidural catheter is placed and a modest morphine infusion begun at 2 mg/hour. She reports a significant drop in her pain levels, now rated to be a 4 or 5 on a scale of 0 to 10. The morphine is titrated upward to 3.5 mg/hour, and she reports excellent relief rated to be a 2 on a scale of 0 to 10. A permanent epidural catheter is placed the following day. Once the initial postoperative discomfort is gone, she is maintained on the 3.5-mg morphine/hour for approximately 2 weeks. She reports increasing pain. A 0.15% solution of bupivacaine is added to the regimen. Her pain relief is again reported to be adequate. Over the next few weeks her pain levels subsequently elevate, and the bupivacaine concentration is increased to 0.25%. Pain relief results, but she reports a feeling of heaviness in her ankles and feet that is very uncomfortable for her. The bupivacaine concentration is titrated downward and the morphine dosage titrated upward. With increasing morphine doses the pain is only reduced to a level of 5 on a scale of 0 to 10. She elects to increase the bupivacaine concentration once again regardless of the heavy feeling in her lower extremities. Her pain relief remains adequate until she dies.

Clinical Accountabilities

1. Assess surgical sequelae and initial response to analgesic therapy:
   - Use a flow sheet to document vital signs, drug and dosage administered, pain level, sedation level.
   - Adverse effects of analgesic therapy: decreased respiratory rate? altered level of consciousness? hypotension? nausea/vomiting? pruritus? urinary retention? numbness, tingling, or heaviness in lower extremities? difficulty in ambulating? Rate and depth of respirations must be carefully monitored.
   - Catheter placement complications: dislodged catheter? leaking catheter? pain when drug is injected into the catheter? fluid accumulation in the pump pocket?

Clinical Accountabilities *(Continued)*

 – Sutures intact? drainage at incision or catheter exit sites? swelling at incision site?
 – Signs of epidural hematoma: intense back pain? rapid onset of leg weakness/spasm? decreased reflexes in lower extremities? loss of bladder/bowel control?
 – Pain: incision pain (procedural pain) versus postoperative pain or pain secondary to chronic disease?

7. Manage adverse side effects by notifying physician and/or initiating protocol: respiratory rate <8, sedation level >2 (0–3 scale), pain rating >4 (0–10 scale), nausea/vomiting, pruritus, urinary retention.

8. Ensure adequate analgesia.
 – Incision pain: common even in the presence of epidural opioids; occurs at exit sites, insertion sites, tunneled catheter pathways, implanted pump pockets; will resolve as tissue heals; treat mild pain with nonopioid analgesics; notify physician for severe pain.
 – Taper systemic opioid dosage while adjusting the spinal analgesic dosage to prevent symptoms of opioid withdrawal for those patients who have been maintained on significant opioid dosages.
 – Administer bolus injections and/or maintain continual infusion for postoperative patients.
 – Titrate epidural continuous infusion per physician's orders/protocol for chronic pain conditions.

9. Provide proper external catheter and wound care:
 – Assess for fluid accumulation in the pump pocket; may occur soon after placement; commonly resolves without treatment.
 – Check dressing for excessive drainage/intactness every 8 hours and as needed.
 – Change dressings at exit site per institutional protocol: sterile dressing changes on the permanent catheter exit site and transparent dressing changes on the temporary catheter exit site (must use extreme caution as catheter is easily dislodged).

Continued on following page

Clinical Accountabilities *(Continued)*

– Cleanse wound, catheter connection sites per protocol with antimicrobial solution. Do not use alcohol.
– Use tubing without injection ports and label "for epidural use only."
– Change 0.22-µ filter and tubing per protocol.

5. Implement appropriate infection control interventions:

– Administer prophylactic antibiotics per institutional protocol.
– Monitor for signs of infection at incision/exit sites (redness, discharge, tenderness, warmth). Treat local infection with careful cleansing and antibiotic ointment.
– Monitor for inflammation along the tunneled catheter path, report to physician, and initiate interventions as ordered.
– Monitor for signs of infection in the epidural space: pain during epidural injections, fluid collection at the posterior incision site, continual back pain, increase in temperature and/or white count; may require epidural aspirate for culture and sensitivity per protocol. Administer parenteral antibiotics for confirmed infection per orders.
– Monitor for signs of infection in the pump pocket: swelling, redness, warmth, and localized pain. Notify physician for further evaluation.

6. Educate patient/family/caregiver on proper catheter and equipment maintenance:

– Use of pain log that documents the level of pain and need for rescue dosing.
– Signs of infection that require physician notification.
– Adverse effects of therapy that require physician notification.
– Exit site care/dressing changes, tubing exchanges.

Clinical Accountabilities *(Continued)*

- External pump maintenance and trouble-shooting.
- Appropriate schedule for internal pump refills/follow-up visits for maintenance.

7. Provide continued outpatient monitoring and maintenance of therapy:
- Pain levels.
- Adverse effects of therapy.
- Patient/family understanding of therapy.

BIBLIOGRAPHY

Ballantyne, J.C., Carr, D.B., Chalmers, T.C., Dear, K.B.G., Angelillo, I.F., & Mosteller, F. (1993). Postoperative patient-controlled analgesia: Meta-analyses of initial randomized control trials. *Journal of Clinical Anesthesiology 5,* 182–193.

Broekema, A.A., Gielen, J.J.M., & Hennis, P.J. (1996). Postoperative analgesia with continuous epidural sufentanil and bupivacaine: A prospective study in 614 patients. *Anesthesia and Analgesia 82,* 754–759.

DeKock, M., Famenne, F., Deckers, G., & Scholtes, J.L. (1995). Epidural clonidine or sufentanil for intraoperative and postoperative analgesia. *Anesthesia and Analgesia 81,* 1154–1162.

DuPen, S.L., & Williams, A.R. (1992). Management of patients receiving combined epidural morphine and bupivacaine for the treatment of cancer pain. *Journal of Pain and Symptom Management 7*(2), 125–127.

Edwards, W.T. (1990). Optimizing opioid treatment of post-operative pain. *Journal of Pain and Symptom Management 5*(1), S24–S36.

Eisenach, J., Detweiler, D., & Hood, D. (1993). Hemodynamic and analgesic actions of epidurally administered clonidine. *Anesthesiology 78*(2), 277–287.

Eisenach, J.C., DuPen, S., Dubois, M., Miguel, R., & Allin, D. (1995). Epidural clonidine for intractable cancer pain. *Pain 61*(3), 391–399.

Grass, J. (1992). Sufentanil: Clinical use as postoperative analgesic-epidural/intrathecal route. *Journal of Pain and Symptom Management 7*(5), 271–286.

Hogan, Q., Haddox, J.D., Abram, S., Weissman, D., Taylor, M.L., & Janjan, N. (1991). Epidural opiates and local anesthetics for the management of cancer pain. *Pain 46*, 271–279.

Krames, E.S. (1993). Intrathecal infusional therapies for intractable pain: Patient management guidelines. *Journal of Pain and Symptom Management 8*(1), 36–46.

Ready, L.B. (1990). Spinal opioids in the management of acute and postoperative pain. *Journal of Pain and Symptom Management 5*, 138–145.

Sabbe, M.B., & Yaksh, T.L. (1990). Pharmacology of spinal opioids. *Journal of Pain and Symptom Management 5*(3), 191–203.

St. Marie, B. (1994). *Management of cancer pain with epidural morphine independent study module.* St. Paul, MN: SIMS Deltec, Inc.

Turnage, G., Clark, L., & Wild, L. (1990). Spinal opioids: A nursing perspective. *Journal of Pain and Symptom Management 5*, 154–162.

6
Physical Modalities

OVERVIEW

Nonpharmacologic interventions form the foundation of chronic pain management and supplement pharmacologic means of relieving acute pain. Although pain relief has commonly been associated with the administration of medications, there is growing understanding and application of physical and psychologic methods that help patients gain control over their pain. These interventions are broadly classified into two categories: (1) **physical modalities** that include both noninvasive and invasive therapies; (2) **cognitive behavioral interventions.**

Noninvasive physical agents are external interventions intended to achieve a specific physiologic response that results in relieving or reducing pain. Application of heat or cold, massage, exercise, and transcutaneous electrical nerve stimulation (TENS) are typical physical agents. Invasive physical therapies include anesthetic and neurosurgical interventions that provide a more permanent analgesic effect.

Reconceptualization of pain is at the center of cognitive-behavioral treatment. Changing beliefs and expectations about pain help patients alter their response to the pain experience. Cognitive-behavioral methods require an internal locus of control because the pain response is determined by the patient's own knowledge and conscious behavior. Education, then, becomes a fundamental building block of cognitive-behavioral interventions and is requisite for success in all pain management situations. A variety of techniques are learned and applied in an effort to manage pain, especially persistent pain. Some examples are distraction, relaxation, imagery, music, and biofeedback. See Chapter 7 for a detailed discussion.

Frequently, multiple interventions are employed.

TABLE 6–1   *Noninvasive Nonpharmacologic Interventions for Pain Management*

PHYSICAL	COGNITIVE BEHAVIORAL
Heat and cold massage	Education
Exercise (movement)	Relaxation
Immobilization	Imagery
TENS	Distraction
Accupressure	Biofeedback
	Music

Adapted from Acute Pain Management Guideline Panel. (1992). Acute Pain Management: *Operative or medical procedures and trauma.* AHCPR Pub. No. 92-0032. Rockville, MD: U.S. Department of Health and Human Services, Agency for Health Care Policy and Research.

Not only are physical and cognitive-behavioral modalities combined, but within each category there may be several beneficial interventions. For example, a single patient may utilize heat, massage and exercise from the noninvasive physical agent group while applying cognitive-behavioral methods, such as music therapy and a variety of relaxation techniques. Choice of nonpharmacologic modalities is highly individualized because an intervention that is successful for one patient may not be effective for another. This is particularly true of the cognitive-behavioral strategies because activities may be associated with past experiences that were either positive or negative. Selection, therefore, is patient dependent and reflects individual variation, experiential bias, and personal preference. Regardless of type, nonpharmacologic modalities support the fundamental principle of pain management— put the patient in control of the pain (Table 6–1).

This chapter focuses on physical modalities while Chapter 7 explores cognitive-behavioral therapies.

NONINVASIVE

Heat and Cold

Heat

An age-old therapy, heat raises the pain threshold through several mechanisms. Muscle spindle excitability decreases, with resultant muscle relaxation and reduced spasm. Heat produces vasodilatation, which decreases congestion in the affected area by facilitating removal of the products of inflammation. Temperature receptors in the skin are affected, and these, in turn, stimulate pain-inhibiting reflexes.

Heat may be classified as dry or moist, superficial or deep. Examples of *dry heat* are heat cradles, goose neck lamps, electric heating pads, or even direct sunlight (using sunscreen, of course). These applications are common because they are easy to use. *Moist heat* includes hot water bottles, hot soaks, baths or showers, hot packs, hydrotherapy, or paraffin baths. All of these measures provide superficial heat, that is, they are based on skin contact. *Deep heat* is produced by shortwave diathermy and ultrasound, methods that require skilled personnel. These heat therapies are designed to penetrate deep body structures, such as joints, tendons, and bone. Pain due to muscle, joint, and soft-tissue pathology is particularly responsive to heat therapy. Low-back pain (due to degenerative joint disease or intervertebral disc disease), painful arthritic joints, and myofibrositis are just a few of the musculoskeletal disorders that may be treated with heat. Gastrointestinal (GI) tract and uterine smooth-musculature spasm are highly responsive to heat. Numerous soft-tissue conditions also benefit from heat therapy.

Like any intervention, however, heat must be used appropriately. There are clinical conditions in which heat is clearly contraindicated. Some of these are acute trauma and/or bleeding (increases tendency to bleed); malignancy site (speeds up growth of malignancy); impaired sensation or anesthetized area (risk of burns); acute stage of rheumatoid arthritis (increases cartilage degeneration); area of decreased vascularity (increased metabolic demand with inadequate oxygenation may cause necrosis). Obtunded patients or those otherwise unable to communicate excessive temperature are not candidates for heat interventions. Temperature guidelines for each type of application are important to prevent burns and to ensure the desired therapeutic effect. Electrical safety is essential when using heating pads or other electrical devices. Diathermy is contraindicated in patients who have pacemakers or metal implants close to the energy source. Although there are exclusions for heat therapy, it remains a solid choice for many pain situations.

Cold

Cold therapy, or *cryotherapy*, reduces muscle tone and slows conduction in the muscle to reduce spasm secondary to underlying joint/skeletal pathology. In physiologic contrast to heat, cold reduces circulation to the area of application, decreasing edema and bleeding. Through an indirect effect on nerve fibers, cold slows nerve conduction, reducing pain sensation.

Ice bags, frozen gel packs (also called cold hydrocollator packs), chemical cold packs, and a variety of improvised cold packs or ice gloves/bags are the usual forms of cold application. Temperature and length of exposure are critical to avoid frostbite/necrosis and to achieve desired therapeutic effect. They differ according to the method used. Consideration must be given to protecting the patient by separating the cold device from the skin with some type of cloth barrier. To reduce cold sensation further, additional layers of cloth may be added.

Cold is the therapy of choice initially (first 48 hours) for trauma (not severe injury) and other acute pain. Pain in trauma, resulting in sprains, cuts, or bruises, can be alleviated or prevented by early cold application. Perception of pain is decreased, as are bleeding and edema formation. These same qualities contribute to the use of cold postoperatively, especially after certain orthopedic procedures. Headaches, dental pain, minor burns, acute calcific bursitis, and early epicondylitis are a few other painful conditions that may be relieved by cold.

Some conditions in which cold is contraindicated are Raynaud's phenomenon; diabetes mellitus and peripheral vascular disease with arterial insufficiency; and cold hypersensitivity. The latter, though rare, may be manifested by urticaria, erythema, itching, and other signs of histamine release. Cold is contraindicated for rheumatic disease (except acute phase of rheumatoid arthritis).

As long as neither therapy is contraindicated, heat and cold may be used intermittently. For some conditions, alternating heat and cold is more effective than one therapy alone (e.g., severe pain). Either heat or cold may be used in other conditions, such as muscle spasm secondary to underlying joint/skeletal pathology. Generally, however, each therapy has particular effectiveness for a given condition. An interesting twist is that acute rheumatoid arthritis responds well to cold and is aggravated by heat; conversely, painful stiff joints of most arthritic conditions are improved by heat and exacerbated by cold. It is important to distinguish appropriate uses for heat or cold and then to respect the patient's individual response to the therapy.

Manual Therapies

Massage

"Massage is the application of touch or force to soft tissues, usually muscles, tendons or ligaments, without causing movement or change in position of a joint" (Haldeman, 1995). An ancient means of relieving pain, massage is a therapeutic intervention that increases circulation and relaxes musculature. When applied to the back, massage can relieve tension throughout the body. The exact mechanism of massage is not clearly understood.

Several considerations may apply, one of them being the time spent personally, quietly with the patient with the "laying on of hands." Massage is a form of therapeutic touch. Therapeutic touch is founded on the energy field theory, which proposes an interconnectedness with others and the environment. Therapeutic touch includes such interventions as meridian tracing, which is the application of light massage at points along an imaginary line on the surface of the body. Meridians are defined in Chinese medicine as the pathways through which the life force or energy flows. Acupressure, too, falls in this category. Also originating with the Chinese, acupressure is based on the "CH'i" and is a circular motion with a finger or knuckle, exerting pressure over one of numerous points along meridians of the body. Endorphin release has been associated with pressure at these points, decreasing pain. These interventions have been particularly successful in relieving tension by relaxing muscles in the head, neck, and shoulder areas. Another therapeutic touch method is reflexology. The theory of reflexology divides the body into ten zones, each zone corresponding to one of the fingers or toes. Massage of the hand or foot, then, is purported to provide analgesia in the corresponding zone. General relaxation has been noted with this method.

The most common form of massage is back massage. Done correctly, back massage relieves tension, relaxes muscles of the back, improves circulation, and reduces edema. Clinicians must not underestimate the power of this very simple technique. In only five minutes of massage, major relaxation can be achieved. Rarely contraindicated, there is no cost involved, and a family member can easily learn the technique. Most people will use the effleurage or light stroking movements using a lotion or oil to lubricate and facilitate the hand movements. Strokes are long, smooth, and gentle, always in the direction of the heart. More sophisticated massage by experienced clinicians may include kneading (pétrissage), connective tissue massage, which is deeper and provides a sensation of warmth, or deep-tissue massage, which is designed to loosen adhesions or mobilize deeper muscles, ligaments, or tendons.

Mobilization and Manipulation

The purpose of mobilization is to stretch muscles and ligaments or move joints to achieve an increased range of motion. One example is stretching the muscle against resistance. Stretching must be done firmly but cautiously to avoid tissue tears. Mobilization and manipulation are similar techniques, the basic difference being that the amount of thrust against joints is greater in manipulation. In addition to possible increase in range of motion, manual therapies increase circulation, reduce edema, and relax muscles. Pain thresholds are increased, though the exact mechanism is not understood. Typically, these therapies are provided by chiropractors, osteopaths, and naturopaths.

Vibration

A little-used intervention that shows potential is vibration, applied to a localized area of discomfort. Vibration provides pain relief by reducing sensation. A numbness occurs to the area that lasts for varying lengths of time. Although vibration is not frequently used in medical regimens, the general population has found value in relief of minor discomforts through handheld or larger devices, pads, or chairs. Devices may be directed over the affected area or next to the area if sensitivity is too great. Usage ranges from relief of muscle spasms and tension to arthritis. Vibration is contraindicated in actual or suspected thrombophlebitis, areas of skin breakdown, or disorders that are aggravated by motion.

Exercise

Therapeutic exercise is believed to relieve pain by improving circulation, reducing edema, and increasing muscle strength and flexibility. A recent theory is that exercise causes the release of endorphins. In addition to the direct effects of exercise, functionality is a major consideration for patients, preserving their ability to perform activities of daily living (ADLs), to return to work, or to maintain an interactive social role.

People give little conscious thought to mobility until it is limited. The action and interaction of muscles and nerves, bones, joints, and ligaments produce locomotion. Disease or trauma often reduces movement either directly because of the underlying pathology or because the patient limits movement to protect against increased pain. In either event, the disuse of muscles, tendons, and ligaments causes loss of strength and further disables the patient. The basic goals of therapeutic exercise are to increase function and reduce pain.

There are several forms of therapeutic exercise. Passive movement occurs when a clinician manually moves a joint or limb. Paralysis and contractures are examples of clinical situations in which passive exercise may be appropriate. Active assisted exercises are those in which the patient's own movement is supplemented either manually or mechanically with special devices. Active exercise is more desirable because the patient voluntarily causes the movement to occur. Caution must be taken to avoid too rigorous exercise in the elderly, as this may cause cardiac complications. Exercise should be stopped if pain occurs in chest or upper extremity as it may signal cardiac involvement. Therapeutic exercise should not be overly aggressive as injuries may occur.

Immobilization

Immobilization may be appropriate in acute situations and is usually implemented to reduce further trauma, bleeding, or edema as well as to provide comfort. Cold may be used concurrently in some cases. When immobilization is used for pain relief, it is a short-term intervention, as opposed to immobilization for treatment of the pathology (e.g., casts, splints, traction). Rest for an affected area is indicated for minor injuries and the acute phase of many musculoskeletal disorders. However, this is time-limited, giving way to the use of other pharmacologic and nonpharmacologic interventions. As noted, exercise is a critical element in restoring and maintaining musculoskeletal strength. Both immobilization and exercise are powerful interventions and must be used appropriately to the situation. Because of this, the degree of mobility in each situation must be clearly defined and not left to chance.

Transcutaneous Electrical Nerve Stimulation (TENS)

Relief of mild to moderate pain can be obtained through the use of **transcutaneous electrical nerve stimulation (TENS).** TENS may also be used adjunctively with other interventions for severe pain. Low-grade electrical current is generated by batteries contained in a small, portable box and conducted by lead wires to electrodes placed on the skin at or near the site of pain. The electrical current crossing the skin between the electrodes stimulates myelinated primary afferent fibers (A fibers) in the dorsal horn of the spinal cord, which in turn inhibit C fibers to block transmission of pain impulses. Other results of localized electrical stimulation include release of endorphins, muscle relaxation, and vasodilation. Approximately 30% of patients with intractable pain can obtain relief for extended periods (Woolf and Thompson, 1995, p. 1191). Although it is effective for either acute or chronic pain, TENS is most often used for chronic pain. The complexity of electrode placement and stimulation may require trial-and-error attempts over time, which is not congruent with the time factor of acute pain. Nor is the need as great in acute pain; pharmacologic and other interventions have proven highly successful in most acute pain situations.

Examples of acute pain relieved by TENS include:

- Postoperative pain (abdominal, thoracic, hip, knee, lower back, and other surgery)
- Sports injuries (e.g., sprains, torn ligaments)
- Fractures (especially fractured ribs)
- Acute arthritis, acute myalgia, myofascial syndrome
- Situations in which opioids are to be avoided (respiratory depression, substance abuse, allergies)

Examples of chronic pain alleviated by TENS include:

- Pain of dysmenorrhea
- Chronic back pain, radiculopathies, compression syndromes
- Neurogenic pain (e.g., peripheral nerve injury, postherpetic neuralgia, trigeminal neuralgia)
- Osteoarthritis
- Phantom limb pain
- Reflex sympathetic dystrophy
- Headache

TENS is designed to relieve pain in a localized area; it is not intended for diffuse pain. Several electrodes may be applied for a large, but contained, site. When TENS is prescribed by a physician, testing its effectiveness is essential. Whether TENS will work, and, if so, what type of TENS should be used is a totally individual matter. To determine whether TENS will be effective for a given patient, a number of attempts may be made to identify precise electrode placement. The type of stimulation also must be matched to patient response; for example, stimulation may be continuous, intermittent (in various patterns), or acupuncture-like. Neither continuous nor intermittent stimulation produces muscle spasm; in contrast, acupuncturelike stimulation elicits small-muscle twitching in specific locations. A major consideration is the patient's ability and desire to comply with the required management of TENS. No therapeutic effect can be obtained for a patient who is unwilling or unable to carry out the appropriate steps for this intervention. Safety, too, dictates that the patient understand and follow directions regarding use (e.g., application to clean/dry skin, removal during bathing or swimming and at bedtime).

The complexity of placement and the skill needed for successful use create some limits for TENS selection, but side effects are minimal: local skin irritation, allergic reaction to one of the components, and occasional equipment failure.

TENS is contraindicated in the following:

- Patients with cardiac pacemakers
- Placement over pregnant uterus
- Placement over broken, irritated skin (burns, wounds, dermatitis, and so on)

Avoid placement:

- Near patient's eyes
- On head or neck if patient has a vascular or seizure disorder

- Over anterior part of neck (risk of causing laryngeal spasm)
- Over carotid sinus or pharyngeal muscle

Use of a TENS unit may preclude more invasive interventions and reduce or eliminate use of opioids. These are compelling reasons to try TENS; however, there are some disadvantages, such as the original cost of the unit and the tendency for decreased effectiveness over time. The latter point is of particular significance to those with chronic pain, although one might argue that the benefits still outweigh the disability associated with intractable pain. TENS presents a viable intervention for pain relief for select patients.

INVASIVE

KEY POINT

Noninvasive treatments should precede invasive approaches.

Invasive nonpharmacologic interventions are used to supplement behavioral, physical, and pharmacologic therapies in selected patient populations. Anesthetic and neurosurgical methods may be indicated to control otherwise intractable acute, cancer, or chronic nonmalignant pain by application of a local anesthetic (LA) or neurolytic agent or by surgical interruption of nerve pathways. Extensive efforts to effectively employ noninvasive methods as well as careful examination of the risks, benefits, and cost of the proposed invasive approach should antedate implementation.

Regional anesthesia is a type of neural blockade that employs a local anesthetic. The local anesthetic agent, when injected at a specific anatomic site, can (1) provide diagnostic information (anatomic source of pain? sympathetic mechanism? somatic or visceral pain? local or referred pain? peripheral or central pain?); (2) furnish prognostic data (assessment of side effects and pain relief likely to result from a planned neurodestructive procedure); (3) be employed prophylactically to prevent sequelae to interventions (delay onset of postoperative pain, decrease complications of postoperative and posttraumatic pain, prevent phantom limb pain and causalgia); and (4) be used therapeutically to provide pain relief.

Common LAs used to provide regional analgesia include procaine, bupivacaine, lidocaine, prilocaine, mepivacaine, tetracaine, and etidocaine. The addition of epinephrine causes local vasoconstriction, thus retarding the drug's absorption from the injection site and reducing the peak blood level. This vasoconstrictive mechanism extends the action of the LA and reduces the risk of systemic toxicity. The addition of corticosteroids seems to stabilize membrane action on nerve fiber endings, as do the LAs, and thus may intensify and lengthen their analgesic action. Some examples of regional anesthesia include:

- Local infiltration of dilute LA for postoperative pain, acute bursitis, tendinitis
- Injection of LA and corticosteroid into trigger points to manage myofascial syndromes
- Intraarticular injection for chronic arthritic pain
- Spinal nerve blocks: occipital nerve block for occipital headache, brachial plexus block for temporary relief following pain or surgery in the upper limb or hand, paravertebral block of the thoracic spinal nerves for rib fractures, sciatic nerve block for pain in the foot, leg, and posterior thigh.
- Sympathetic nervous system blocks for reflex sympathetic dystrophy or peripheral vascular disease

Therapeutic injections of a local anesthetic may provide analgesia that outlives its pharmacologic action. Although pain relief may quickly follow the procedure, the duration of effect is variable and may be only hours to weeks. Results of the neural block may need to be supplemented by other analgesic measures when used to treat acute pain (e.g., opioid analgesics on an as-needed basis), but the dosage of the supplemental analgesic should be markedly smaller postprocedure. When used to treat chronic pain of a complex nature, the neural blockade's therapeutic position is limited (i.e., the extent of the pain may exceed the anatomic distribution of the block and should be seen in the context of a multimodal rehabilitation program).

Neurolysis, a second type of nerve block, employs chemical agents to destroy nerve cell bodies to produce prolonged interference of the transmission of the pain signal. This technique should be reserved for situations in which more conservative strategies have been ineffective. The primary indication is to manage chronic cancer pain. Prior to neurolysis the identified anatomic site is injected with a "test dose" of local anesthetic to ensure that the more permanent blockade will produce pain relief.

After it is determined that a neural blockade has the potential for therapeutic efficacy based on the results of local anesthetic injections, a neurolytic agent (alcohol or phenol) is injected. Alcohol, the classic neurolytic agent, destroys nerve fibers. It triggers intense burning and should be immediately followed by a local anesthetic injection. Phenol, which also is neurodestructive, causes warmth followed by numbness. Neurolytic agents injected around or into a nerve produce pathophysiologic changes of varying degrees and cause temporary or permanent nerve cell body destruction. Examples of neurolytic procedures include:

- Ganglion block for trigeminal neuralgia
- Subarachnoid alcohol or intrathecal phenol injections to relieve cancer pain
- Epidural phenol for cancer pain
- Celiac plexus block to relieve pancreatic cancer pain or severe, chronic visceral pain
- Lumbar sympathetic blocks for chronic painful conditions in the lower limbs

Patients may experience complete relief after a neurolytic procedure. If they have been on chronic opioid therapy, it is imperative to titrate the dosage downward to prevent withdrawal symptoms. In addition, the sudden cessation of pain might also eliminate the stimulating effect of the pain on respiratory effort, and patients could develop respiratory depression. This procedure requires close monitoring and appropriate intervention.

Neurosurgical procedures also are reserved for those for whom every possible less invasive method has been tried without success. Neurodestructive operations may indeed be indicated for those with a life-threatening malignancy and severe, intractable pain. Stereotaxic procedures have been developed that interrupt specific and diffuse pain pathways at specific sites, and the use of controlled radiofrequency current can generate a thermally destructive lesion. These refined techniques allow for discrete lesions with a needle versus a more extensive surgical procedure. A surgical neurectomy involves resection of part of the nerve/nerve root/nerve tract complex and may provide complete anesthesia in the area of the resectioned nerve. Depending on the clinical setting and nature of the pathophysiology, the risks include new pain symptoms as a result of nerve damage at the incisional site or from the nerve division itself, return of pain after transient relief, and postoperative neurologic impairment. These must all be balanced against the proposed, but not guaranteed, advantage of partial or complete pain relief.

The noninvasive physical modalities may provide only temporary relief, but they do have real analgesic efficacy and may be employed in a multitude of settings with a minimum amount of training and/or skills needed. They generally are inexpensive, patient controlled and directed, and universally seen as helpful adjunctive treatment. The invasive therapies are, on the other hand, far more complex procedures requiring considerable expertise and resources. As stated, they are reserved for intractable pain that has not responded to any other intervention and are not to be considered first-line choices for the relief of chronic pain.

BIBLIOGRAPHY

Acute Pain Management Guideline Panel. (1992). *Acute pain management: Operative or medical procedures and trauma.* Clinical practice guideline. AHCPR Pub. No. 92-0032. Rockville, MD.: Agency for Health Care Policy and Research, Public Health Service, U.S. Department of Health and Human Services.

Bonica, J.J., & Buckley, F.P. (1990). Regional analgesia with local anesthetics. In J.J. Bonica (Ed.), *The management of pain* (2nd ed., pp. 1883–1996). Philadelphia: Lea & Febiger.

Bonica, J.J., Buckley, F.P., Moricca, G., & Murphy, T.M. (1990). Neurolytic blockade and hypophysectomy. In J.J. Bonica (Ed.), *The management of pain* (2nd ed., pp. 1980–2043). Philadelphia: Lea & Febiger.

Clinical Practice Guidelines. (1992). *Acute pain management: Operative or medical procedures and trauma.* Rockville, MD: U.S. Department of Health and Human Services: Agency for Health Care Policy and Research.

Haldeman, S. (1995). Manipulation and massage for the relief of back pain. In Wall, P., & Melzack, R. (Eds.), *Textbook of pain* (pp. 1251–1260). New York: Churchill Livingstone.

McCaffery, M. (1979). *Nursing management of the patient with pain.* Philadelphia: Lippincott.

McCaffery, M., & Beebe, A. (1989). *Pain: Clinical manual for nursing practice.* St. Louis: Mosby.

Macrae, J.A. (1987). Therapeutic touch: A practical guide. New York: Knopf.

Nursing Now: Pain. (1985). Nursing '85 Books. Pennsylvania: Springhouse.

Owens, M., & Ehrenreich, D. (1991). Application of nonpharmacologic methods of managing chronic pain. *Holistic Nursing Practice, 6*(1), 32–40.

Watt-Watson, J., & Donovan, M. (1992). *Pain management nursing perspective.* St. Louis: Mosby Year Book.

Woolf, C., & Thompson, J. (1995). Stimulation-induced analgesia: transcutaneous electrical nerve stimulation (TENS) and vibration. In Wall, P., & Melzack, R. (Eds.), *Textbook of pain* (pp. 1191–1205). New York: Churchill Livingstone.

7
Cognitive-Behavioral Therapy

OVERVIEW

The premise of **cognitive-behavioral approaches** is that pain is more than a sensory event: the experience includes cognitive, affective, and behavioral components. Unlike medications or physical agents, cognitive-behavioral approaches do not directly relieve pain; they enable the patient to assume an active role in controlling pain. The goal of therapy is to improve quality of life by changing the way the patient perceives and responds to pain.

Cognitive strategies may be effectively utilized for either acute or chronic pain relief. Basic techniques are essentially the same for each, but time and patient expectations differ. The patient in acute pain is sustained by the time limitations of the experience, the projected end point. "Tomorrow will be better," "Next week I will have only residual discomfort," "Six weeks from now I will not hurt." Such thoughts generate energy and a means of coping with the present. The clinician can build on this momentum by giving the patient tools to alleviate discomfort. Whenever possible, teaching should precede the pain experience. For example, patients should be thoroughly educated prior to surgery or other painful procedures on what to expect and how to manage their experience. That is the ideal time to explore the patient's comfort with various techniques and develop basic skill at one or more of them. When the pain episode is unanticipated, the clinician will have a greater challenge. The teaching must still be done, but the patient's readiness to hear and respond will need to be carefully assessed. A basic principle is to medicate or otherwise make the patient as comfortable as possible before attempting to convey information or share pain-relieving techniques. This practice will enhance the patient's ability to concentrate and retain the learning. A few brief moments in which the patient learns some distraction techniques or relaxation steps may provide valuable resource for controlling the pain experience.

In contrast, chronic pain sufferers feel less control and fear the future as an extension of existing pain, or worse. Their perceptions are based on the negative conditioning of past failures, and that reality is difficult to overcome. Yet it is the patient with prolonged unrelieved pain who most needs to apply cognitive-behavioral strategies.

Patients with chronic pain commonly exhibit a predictable pattern of response. Over time, as the pain becomes more dominant in their lives, patients become increasingly fearful and victimized by their own suffering. Behaviors are reactive, defensive to avoid additional hurt. Pain centers the patient's attention inward, and activities follow the pain dictate. The patient may remain in bed or sit for long periods, avoiding movement because of the discomfort associated with activity. Progressive deterioration follows as muscle strength, joint mobility, and tendon flexibility are decreased. Limited mobility then begins to restrict social interactions, leaving the patient with less distractions from self. Soon there is little to do and little else to think about. There is only pain.

In such situations, pain is the controller. Pain determines activity. Pain determines socialization. Pain determines one's whole life. Cognitive-behavioral approaches purposefully disrupt such negative cycles and help patients restructure their thinking about their pain and themselves. To accomplish this change, the patient must begin to view pain as manageable and learn ways to intercede, to develop adaptive behaviors. Like most problems in life, looking at the problem in total is overwhelming and seldom leads to concrete action in itself. The solution is to identify single aspects of the whole and address each. For example, patients must consider what triggers pain for them and exert control by avoiding or limiting those factors. Likewise, those activities or stimuli that contribute to relaxation and pain reduction also must be identified and valued.

Patients must examine their family interactions and project reasonable role expectations for themselves. This is, perhaps, the single most important step, the moment of truth for the individual. The patient's ability to face and to commit to making necessary lifestyle/behavioral changes is the singular determinant of success in chronic pain management.

As patients become more realistic and decisive about their lives, they begin to build greater self-esteem, expand their capacity to learn, and apply techniques that reduce pain and make the experience more tolerable. As each matter is resolved, a pattern of success emerges. For the patient with intractable pain, these may be the first victories ever sustained in the pain battle. The clinician is a critical partner in assisting this process. Reconceptualization includes modification of thoughts and beliefs about pain and development of a satisfying, albeit a redesigned, self-image. Behavior changes follow restructured thinking. The patient becomes resourceful rather than helpless.

Active participation is the critical element. This demands a commitment on the part of the patient, faith in themselves, and trust in the clinician. During the initial period, antidepressants, anxiolytics, more potent analgesics, or combinations of medications may be used to support the patient's immediate needs. These are assistive measures rather than long-term therapies. The rationale follows Maslow's hierarchy of needs (i.e., the patient cannot be expected to learn while in extreme need). Support is essential to patients who often are frail in the face of pain; however, no amount of intervention by any health care worker alone can attain the goal, because the goal is personal control.

"Sick" or maladaptive behaviors, such as a sedentary lifestyle, reliance on medications and dependence on others, are converted to positive, adaptive behaviors that enhance health and quality of life. This transformation may be evident in a number of ways: physical conditioning through exercise; personal control of influences on pain; and medication reduction and decreased dependence on the health care system (fewer hospitalizations, physician office visits, etc.). This conversion begins with reconceptualization of pain and self and progresses through learning and adapting specific pain relief techniques that will be described.

MOST COMMON TECHNIQUES

Education

Information is power. Sharing information with patients gives them power and control over their experience and can positively affect outcomes. **Education** is a basic component of patient care that should have equal value with the most sophisticated, state-of-the-art interventions. Scientific breakthroughs were never intended to replace fundamentals, but to augment them. For example, administration of the most potent antimicrobials for infection is not a substitute for simple handwashing. Analgesics and education can be similarly compared in the pain situation. The action of an analgesic, though very beneficial, is not intended to replace teaching the patient how to cope with the pain.

Education alleviates fear by making the unknown known. Most people can cope with situations when they understand what is happening. The unknown conjures up mental pictures that are inaccurate and far worse than any reality. Fear of the unknown causes tension and a lowered pain threshold; conversely, knowledge fosters composure and a sense of order even when there is discomfort.

In addition to providing psychologic well-being, education is essential to speed up physical recovery. The typical example is teaching patients prior to surgery the activities that will be expected postoperatively. Coughing, deep breathing, turning, walking are uncomfortable and, without education, would certainly be avoided. By understanding the value of these activities, the patient makes a conscious decision to endure temporary discomfort to facilitate healing. For those with chronic pain, the present discomfort may be the price a patient is willing to pay for greater functionality or a more tolerable level of pain for the long term. Thus, the patient becomes an active partner in his or her own treatment and recovery.

Patients deserve to understand what is happening to their bodies, both the pathology and any procedures that are imposed for diagnostic or therapeutic purposes. When pain is part of the clinical picture, the patient also needs to know specific ways to manage the pain. Active participation promotes the effectiveness of medications or other treatments and becomes part of the therapy itself. Studies with surgical patients have shown that those who had thorough preoperative teaching required less analgesics and had a shorter, better postoperative course than those with less extensive preparation. To provide quality care, the clinician is bound to teach as well as treat patients. Education is the first step toward putting patients in control of their pain because understanding removes fear and opens possibilities.

Distraction

Distraction is a simple technique that people use all the time without conscious thought. The basis of distraction is the refocusing of attention away from the pain experience (McCaffery & Beebe, 1989). A wide range of distractors may need to be introduced to dull awareness of pain, the choice being limited only by the physical surroundings and patient preference. Counting various items, reading, watching television, playing computer games, reciting poetry or limericks, rhythmic breathing, engaging in hobbies are only a few of the potential activities a patient may choose.

A great advantage is that most patients can practice distraction with minimal assist initially. Children (old enough to understand and follow directions) through the elderly can participate in this technique. The acute pain of procedures can be made more bearable when the patient practices distraction during the process. Yet, chronic pain patients, too, can benefit from distraction techniques. Although the pain is prolonged, multiple and more complex activities can maintain a level of pain tolerance that may sustain the patient throughout much of the day. Distraction is a no-cost, highly flexible technique that can be applied at any time and under the full control of the patient.

On the down side, the patient may be fatigued and more acutely aware of the pain after such an exercise.

This occurs because of the intense concentration that is inherent in the technique. Another disadvantage is that others may not believe the patient has real pain. Such misconceptions are due to lack of understanding of this strategy and the superficial observation that the patient appears to be comfortable while employing distraction.

Some general guidelines are:

- Use pleasurable stimuli/activities.
- Match the distractor to the person and situation.
- Medicate the patient as usual; distraction does not eliminate pain, it makes pain more tolerable.
- Let the patient take charge.
- Encourage practice.

Distraction is a powerful, yet simple, technique. All patients experiencing pain should have the opportunity to learn and apply distraction. The more "tools" the patient has available to use in the control of pain, the more effective and independent he or she will be.

Relaxation

Anxiety, just like fear, causes muscle tension and increased sympathetic nervous system activity ("fight or flight response"). Blood pressure rises, the pulse quickens, and respirations become more rapid. The person is in a heightened state of tension, both mentally and physically. As anxiety intensifies, tolerance to pain decreases and patients become trapped in the cycle of anxiety and pain.

Relaxation, described as a state of relative freedom from anxiety and tension, produces a physical and emotional state opposite to that of anxiety. Physiologically, relaxation produces lower blood pressure, decreased pulse, respirations, and muscle tone and a general sense of tranquility. In such a state, pain is usually more tolerable. It is obvious, then, that techniques to induce relaxation assist in breaking the anxiety/pain cycle and are supplemental tools in pain management.

Telling a patient to relax does not make it happen; on the contrary, the stress caused by making such a statement may actually increase anxiety and tension. Patients need to understand the relationship between relaxation and pain reduction, then learn and practice techniques. There are a wide variety of approaches to relaxation, including meditation, progressive muscle relaxation, rhythmic breathing, and autogenic relaxation training. Imagery, biofeedback, and hypnosis/self-hypnosis are discussed separately here for simplicity, but all have commonalities and overlap for relaxation response.

"**Meditation** is a continuous stream of effortless concentration, on a single point, over an extended period of time" (Nuernberger, 1990). The relationship between relaxation and meditation is a fluid one in which meditation cannot be achieved without a relaxed state, yet meditation produces relaxation. As defined, meditation may include diverse practices ranging from simple transcendental meditation to the centuries-old methods of the Zen or Hindu religions or yoga (which also consists of gentle exercises). The clinician may refer the patient for more in-depth meditation training or may seek resources to teach some basic meditation techniques in the clinical setting. Resources may include tapes or written material that the patient or clinician may use in this effort. Patients can readily learn meditation techniques, especially some of the simplest ones that facilitate concentration. An example of simple relaxation would be assuming a comfortable upright position in a quiet environment free of distractions, closing the eyes, and doing breathing exercises to promote relaxation. When the body has begun to relax, the patient exclusively focuses on a single wish or thought. Initially such concentration, if fully attained, will last only 2 to 3 minutes. Further development will result in more skillful, longer-lasting meditation that can be done daily.

Progressive muscle relaxation (PMR) refers to exercises in which the patient alternately tenses and relaxes muscle groups. For example, the patient will tense or flex the muscles of the fingers, hand, forearm, and so on in a sequential manner. As a group of muscles are tensed, the patient will hold that tension for a few seconds, then relax those muscles and focus on the difference in the two feelings, "experiencing" the feeling of relaxation. These exercises continue until they have been done with all the muscle groups in the body. By completion, the patient should be in a fully relaxed state. The concept of tension/relaxation of muscles can be modified in a number of different exercises. Shorter exercises may be of value for more immediate responses.

A common and easily applied technique is that of rhythmic, diaphragmatic breathing. The patient is taught to do abdominal breathing, which is natural to infants. Using the diaphragm, the patient inhales and exhales, counting to create a soft rhythmic pattern. The patient concentrates on relaxing with exhalation, feeling the tension leave the body with the exhaled air. As with previous techniques, there are tapes available to assist the patient with mastering this technique. This technique may be used for acute or chronic pain and has been used successfully in relaxation during the first stage of labor.

Autogenic training is a self-suggestion technique in which the patient silently repeats phrases that denote physical relaxation about various body parts. "My left leg feels heavy," "My right arm feels warm" are some examples. The repetition, the relaxation content, and the focus on a specific area of the body all contribute to reinforcing a positive feeling in the patient. There are many variations of this technique. Autogenic training may be used alone or with other techniques.

Biofeedback

Biofeedback is giving a person information about his or her own physiologic functions so that he or she can control that function. This is a more complex technique that is not practiced by the clinician working in most settings; however, knowledge of this technique and the ability to identify pain clinics or other centers for referral are important. Skin temperature (relative to vascular system changes), skin resistance, muscle tension, pulse volume, brain waves can be monitored and communicated to the patient in a variety of ways.

An example is electromyogram (EMG) biofeedback, which reads electrical activity in a muscle and converts that reading to a beeping tone that increases or decreases in pitch and speed in response to the corresponding increase or decrease in muscle tension. By receiving the information of muscle tension via the beeping tone, the patient is able to voluntarily relax the affected muscles. The beeping tone gives continual feedback about the effectiveness of actions, thereby providing positive reinforcement of desired behavior. It should be noted that biofeedback, although it technically is information sharing, depends on some action by the patient to produce an improved outcome. It is at this point that the patient may apply one or more of the relaxation techniques mentioned, frequently autogenic training. Biofeedback techniques have been useful in some patients with Raynaud's disease, reflex sympathetic dystrophy, back and neck pain, phantom-limb pain, and muscle contraction headaches. More controlled studies are necessary about this relatively recent technique.

Hypnosis

Hypnosis is a state of relaxation in which a person's attention is intensely focused and that person is highly receptive to suggestions by the therapist. Contrary to common belief, hypnosis does not put the subject to sleep; the subject is a consenting, active participant. Nor is the patient weak or passive when responding to hypnosis; on the contrary, suggestibility is thought to be related to the subject's belief in hypnosis and determination to facilitate the desired outcome. Thus, effectiveness depends on both the skill of the therapist and the commitment and trust of the patient. Suggestions made while in this highly receptive state may produce reduced or altered pain perception after the hypnosis. The mechanism of hypnosis is not clearly understood, yet there is anecdotal evidence of effectiveness in some situations. Hypnosis must be conducted or taught by a trained specialist. Although usually guided by a specialist, patients can, with considerable practice, be taught to induce a hypnotic-like state themselves. This is possible due to the active participation and fierce concentration that such patients exhibit. Hypnosis is not as commonly used as the other cognitive-behavioral techniques, but it has a place in certain situations.

Imagery

Everyone has practiced imagery in the form of daydreaming or reminiscing. Like other cognitive techniques, imagery is really an extension of normal behaviors. **Imagery** is a form of relaxation that dulls awareness of reality and creates a daydream state that focuses on mental images. The patient is fully awake, but attention is deflected from pain and other stimuli and concentrated on pleasant thoughts. The reader will note the similarities and overlap that occur between techniques previously discussed. There is an element of distraction in imagery (i.e., attention is diverted from thought of pain). As in hypnosis, the patient focuses attention intensely, although in imagery the focus is on pleasant mental images. For imagery, like meditation or other techniques, initial relaxation is often preceded by simple relaxation techniques, such as breathing exercises or progressive muscle relaxation. There are distinctions between techniques, yet they all foster self-control, and all produce some level of relaxation.

The term *guided imagery* refers to the intentional use of imagery for a therapeutic effect. Breaking the anxiety and pain cycle with relaxation and imagery is a powerful adjunct to other pain interventions. Images may take the shape of warm memories or wishful events. Sometimes they are very simple, visualizing a pleasant scene; at other times they can be very intense, involving more senses than just vision (e.g., smell, touch, taste, hearing). According to McCaffery (1979, p. 156), the more senses are used in imagery, the more effective the results that may be obtained. Patients who become deeply engrossed in their imagery are likely to experience a deeper state of relaxation. In summarizing research on relief of cancer pain, Sloman points out that guided imagery produces "clinically significant reduction in the experience of pain and noxious sensations" (1995, p. 699). Imagery is relatively easy for patients to learn, and clinicians can assist by suggesting pleasant mental pictures for thought. Tapes and guidelines are available to give more specific instructions and facilitate learning for patients and families.

Music

Music has been called a universal language because it reaches people of all ages and backgrounds. It is hardly possible to spend a day without some music, whether on the radio or television or in an elevator, office, or store or even waiting on the phone. More specifically, music is selected and played by individuals to create relaxation, enlivenment, or other emotional satisfaction. People accept music as a part of the fabric of their lives. It is not surprising, then, that music is an acceptable and pleasurable intervention when used appropriately.

The therapeutic effect of music has been supported by scientific studies. Research has demonstrated that soothing music produces relaxation, as evidenced by such physiologic responses as decreased blood pressure, heart rate, respirations, blood levels of adrenocorticotropic hormone (ACTH), muscle tone, and oxygen consumption and metabolic rates, and increased release of endorphins and induced sleep. In a study of preterm infants, music was shown to be effective in "reducing stress-related responses to noxious interventions" (Burke et al., 1995). Kaminski and Hall (1996, pp. 46–47) relate the sedative effects of soothing music on neonates (decreased motor activity, grimacing, crying) and fetuses (decreased fetal movement). These studies demonstrate the human response to music without regard to age or other personal characteristics. Music has been successfully used to increase pain thresholds and improve emotional state in a variety of situations involving both acute and chronic pain.

Like the other cognitive-behavioral techniques discussed, music produces relaxation in several overlapping ways. In the simplest sense, music causes attention to be distracted away from the pain focus. Imagery and music often are partners, as music stirs emotions that then can translate into pleasant images that reinforce the heightened concentration state. At another, more primitive and subconscious level, the rhythm and harmony of the music may determine human beings' perception of and response to their environment. Schorr writes that "music as patterned environmental resonance influences the interconnectedness of the entire living system" (1993, p. 81).

In using or recommending music therapeutically to reduce pain perception, the clinician must remember some basic guidelines:

- Music should be soothing (about 60–72 beats/minute).
- Music should be familiar to the patient (inability to predict the stimuli can increase anxiety).
- The patient must be willing to listen to the music (patients who do not desire music will experience increased tension).
- Selection of music should be left to the patient (individual preference varies; results are best with personalized choice).
- The patient should control the volume.
- Whenever possible, headphones are recommended because they block out other, noxious sounds.

Music is an easy and pleasurable technique for decreasing pain perception and inducing relaxation. For hospitalized or isolated patients, music provides a link with their identity, stimulates memories, and fills a void. Patients can release tension with music and through selection and voluntary use of music exert control over their pain.

The first and critical step in cognitive-behavioral therapy is the reconceptualization of pain by the patient; that is, the patient must believe that the pain is manageable and more specifically that she or he can control the pain. Cognitive-behavioral techniques are powerful adjuncts to other pain relief interventions. As extensions of normal behavior, these techniques are relatively simple to learn and generally cost little or nothing. The patient becomes an active participant in controlling pain. The techniques described, as well as those yet to come (e.g., aroma therapy), form the new frontier for altered pain perception.

BIBLIOGRAPHY

Burke, M., Walsh, J., Oehler, J., & Gingras, J. (1995). Music therapy following suctioning: Four case studies. *Neonatal Network, 14*(7), 41–49.

Davenport, L. (1996). Guided Imagery Gets Respect. *Healthcare Forum Journal,* Nov./Dec., 28–32.

Jessup, B., & Gallegos, X. (1995). Relaxation and biofeedback. In Wall, P., & Melzack, R. (Eds.), *Textbook of pain.* (pp. 1321–1332). New York: Churchill Livingstone.

Kaminski, J., & Hall, W. (1996). The effect of soothing music on neonatal behavioral states in the hospital newborn nursery. *Neonatal Network, 24*(1), 45–52.

Keefe, R., Beauprè, P., Weiner, D., & Siegler, I. (1996). Pain in older adults: A cognitive-behavioral perspective. In Ferrell, B.R., & Ferrell, B.A. (Eds.), *Pain in the elderly.* (pp. 11–19). Seattle: IASP Press.

Lane, D. (1992). Music therapy: A gift beyond measure. *Oncology Nursing Forum, 19*(6), 863–867.

McCaffery, M. (1979). *Nursing management of the patient with pain.* Philadelphia: Lippincott.

McCaffery, M., & Beebe, A. (1989). *Pain: Clinical manual for nursing practice.* St. Louis: Mosby.

Nuernberger, P. (1990). *Freedom from stress: A holistic approach.* Himalayan International Institute of Yoga Science and Philosophy Publishers.

Palakanis, K., DeNobile, J., Sweeney, W., & Blankenship, C. (1994). Effect of music therapy on state anxiety in patients undergoing flexible sigmoidoscopy. *Diseases of the Colon & Rectum, 37*(5), 478–481.

Schorr, J.A. (1993). Music and pattern change in chronic pain. *Advances in Nursing Science,* 17–36.

Sloman, R. (1995). Relaxation and the relief of cancer pain. *Nursing Clinics of North America, 30*(4), 697–709.

Turk, D., & Meichenbaum, D. (1995). A cognitive-behavioral approach to pain management. In Wall, P., & Melzack, R. (Eds.), *Textbook of pain,* (pp. 1337–1347). New York: Churchill Livingstone.

Watt-Watson, J., & Donovan, M. (1992). *Pain management nursing perspective.* St. Louis: Mosby Year Book.

8
Acute Pain

There are many ways to classify the pain experience. The most basic and perhaps simplest division categorizes pain as acute or chronic. This categorization focuses on the etiology and expected trajectory of the pain experience.

The pathophysiology of **acute pain** is fairly well understood, diagnosis is rarely difficult, and therapy is generally effective. Given the effectiveness of the therapy and the self-limiting nature of the disease or injury, pain usually abates in a matter of days or weeks. However, untreated or undertreated pain can cause a "heightened awareness" at peripheral pain receptors and increased sensory input at the spinal cord level. This results in less efficient and more difficult pain management. As will be seen, acute pain management with its short-term focus employs different management strategies from those used in managing chronic malignant and nonmalignant pain.

Acute pain can be characterized as follows:

- Precipitating event (injury to the body) with well-defined pattern of onset
- Evidence of tissue damage
- Short-term, usually self-limited
- Progressive resolution within an expected time frame as the tissue heals
- Normal defense mechanism that brings attention to the underlying problem
- Common physiologic responses associated with autonomic nervous system activity: elevated pulse and blood pressure, diaphoresis, and pallor
- Common behavioral responses: grimacing, guarding, verbal expressions of pain

Acute pain from surgery, diagnostic procedures, burns, and trauma is underestimated and under-treated. There are more than 23 million operations (1.5 million in children) performed every year in the United States. Clinical surveys suggest that intramuscular injections on an as-needed basis are inadequate for approximately 50% of postoperative patients, yet this continues to be a commonly ordered intervention. When acute pain is unrelieved, it can lead to postsurgical blood clots, heart attacks, pneumonias, and other physical problems. Resultant behavioral changes can include withdrawal from interpersonal contact and increased sensitivity to external stimuli such as light and sound. Acute pain can contribute to delirium in the intensive care unit. Lack of relief can delay hospital discharge, impede recuperation and recovery, and contribute to psychologic complications (American Pain Society, 1992).

A survey of teaching and community hospitals and some 500 adult participants (Warfield & Kahn, 1995) examined attitudes about acute pain and institutional commitment to the management of acute pain. Less than 50% of the hospitals surveyed had acute pain management programs, but of greater interest was the consumer's attitude toward acute (most likely postoperative) pain management. The majority of patients facing surgery identified their greatest fear as pain that would follow the operative procedure. Eighty percent of the patients reported moderate to extreme pain. Almost three-quarters of the respondents continued to experience pain after receiving pain medication. The problem has been identified, and the therapeutic interventions are readily available. The Agency for Health Care Policy and Research clinical practice guidelines on the management of acute pain (Acute Pain Management Guideline-Panel, 1992) has provided clinicians with a well-researched and comprehensive approach to this very real problem. This chapter is intended to provide the clinician with an overview of the issues.

When the etiology of acute pain is uncertain, rapid diagnosis is a priority. Clinicians should provide symptomatic treatment of the pain while the diagnostic workup is in process. Deferring pain relief until the diagnosis is made is rarely justified. Patients who are comfortable during the diagnostic procedure are better able to cooperate and more likely to trust the health care team members. Initial examination of the acute abdomen could be considered an exception to this approach.

Although acute pain control options may include cognitive-behavioral interventions (e.g., relaxation, imagery), physical agents (e.g., massage, application of heat and/or cold), electroanalgesia (TENS unit), or neural blockade (e.g., intercostal nerve block), they are not substitutes for the pharmacologic management of moderate to severe pain. In fact, most postoperative and trauma pain is preventable or controllable with the use of analgesic agents.

MANAGEMENT PRINCIPLES

The following principles are applicable for all types of acute pain. Drug choice and route, dosage, and scheduling depend on the nature and intensity of the pain. For example, as the tissue heals and the pain resolves, an oral analgesic taken on an as-needed basis can replace the need for scheduled doses of a parenteral opioid. The evaluation of acute pain relies on basic assessment principles (see Chapter 3). The underlying premise is that assessment should be frequent and simple and rely on the patient's self-report. Each instance of unexpected, intense pain needs to be evaluated, especially if it is accompanied by altered vital signs or oliguria.

Choose the Appropriate Drug

The pharmacologic management of mild to moderate pain should begin with a nonopioid analgesic. Acetaminophen, aspirin and other salicylates, and nonsteroidal antiinflammatory drugs (NSAIDs) can be very useful in managing acute pain. Unless NSAIDs are contraindicated, they should be routinely considered. Although postoperative and trauma patients commonly may have nothing by mouth during the immediate acute period, ketorolac (Toradol®), an

NSAID available in parenteral form, may be administered intramuscularly or intravenously. When non-opioids are ineffective as single agents, they may demonstrate an opioid dose-sparing effect when given in combination with an opioid analgesic. See Chapter 4 for more detailed information on pharmacologic agents.

When the maximum dosage of a nonopioid analgesic provides inadequate pain relief, an opioid analgesic should be added to the regimen. Opioid analgesics commonly used for mild to moderate pain include codeine (e.g., Tylenol #3®), oxycodone (e.g., Percocet®), propoxyphene (e.g., Darvocet®), and hydrocodone (e.g., Vicodin®). They are available in low-dose preparations as sole agents or in combination with non-opioid analgesics.

Moderately severe to severe pain should be treated initially with an opioid analgesic. Opioid analgesics are the cornerstone of burn pain, postoperative, and posttraumatic analgesic regimens. Dosage, schedule, incidence and intensity of side effects, and treatment setting are important variables to be considered. Morphine, meperidine (Demerol®), and hydromorphone (Dilaudid®) are commonly selected agents.

Establish an Adequate Dosage That Produces Relief as Quickly and Consistently as Possible

First, provide a suitable initial dose. Because analgesic requirements vary markedly from patient to patient, it is essential to determine the appropriate dose individually. Administer as a one-time dose enough analgesic to make the patient comfortable. Failure to front-load in the presence of severe pain delays adequate relief even though the patient may receive several as-needed or scheduled analgesic doses. A serum drug concentration threshold adequate for relief can be established by administering the analgesic in small increments until the patient reports relief. This measured approach ensures patient safety and comfort by providing enough analgesic for pain relief while avoiding the respiratory depressive effects of overdosing.

Provide enough analgesic to relieve the pain consistently. An analgesic dosage that does not provide adequate relief before it is scheduled to be given again needs to be adjusted. Patient report of inadequacy is considered a valid parameter for titration. It is rare for opioid tolerance or physical dependence to develop with short-term use in opioid-naive patients. If increasing opioid doses are ineffective, there may be residual pathology or a neuropathic component to the pain experience. It is important to remember that patients who have previously received opioid analgesics or who have a history of prior or concurrent substance abuse disorder will require higher initial and maintenance doses, report higher pain scores, and are less likely to experience pruritus and emesis secondary to opioid therapy.

Taper the dosage as the pain decreases. As the tissue heals, the pain intensity lessens. Both dosage and scheduling requirements may change. An expected limited-duration "chronic" pain state postoperatively or posttraumatically may be treated with scheduled analgesics for 36 to 48 hours or longer depending on the nature and severity of the pain. The dosage may be decreased or the schedule changed to an as-needed administration as the pain levels recede.

Schedule Analgesics Appropriately

Base administration schedule on the known half-life of the drug. Each analgesic has an expected period of effectiveness. Scheduling (either as needed or around the clock) should be determined by the duration of the medication's analgesic action. When an analgesic is given with proper timing to prevent pain recurrence, fear and anxiety can be decreased, the pain threshold elevated, relief provided at a decreased dosage, and activity increased. The patient spends less time in pain and can focus resources on restorative activity.

Maintain consistent relief. Pain that is moderate to severe in nature and expected to continue for an identified time should be treated on a scheduled basis. This preventative approach requires that the analgesic be given before pain occurs or increases in intensity. If there is respiratory depression (usually fewer than 8 breaths a minute) or the patient is excessively drowsy, the opioid should be withheld and subsequent dosages reduced. As tissue heals and pain decreases in intensity, as-needed dosing is acceptable.

Choose the Appropriate Route

Consider the immediacy of the need. Outside of spinal analgesia, the intravenous administration of analgesics provides the highest level of relief with the most rapid onset of action. Moderate to severe pain responds most immediately to the intravenous route and is preferable when the patient is unable to take oral medications. All routes other than the intravenous one require a lag time for absorption into the circulation. The intramuscular route has the disadvantage not only of wide fluctuations in absorption, but also of a 30- to 60-minute lag time to peak effect. Spinal analgesia via an epidural opioid and/or local anesthetic is appropriate for identified patient populations. Analgesic onset is rapid and can be very efficacious, but it is not a typical choice for postoperative patients. See Chapter 5 for more detail on intraspinal analgesia for both acute and chronic pain.

Assess the patient's tolerance of the route. Repeated intramuscular injections can cause pain and trauma and deter patients from requesting pain medication. Nausea and/or vomiting or a sore throat or nothing by mouth status may rule out the oral route, but it is important to remember that oral administration is convenient, inexpensive, and appropriate when tolerated. A wide variety of oral nonopioid and opioid analgesics are available.

When changing the route of administration, use appropriate equianalgesic conversion data. Sound knowledge of equianalgesic doses provides safe and effective medication adjustments. Oral analgesics pass from the stomach through the small bowel and then into the portal circulation. They subsequently undergo hepatic metabolism, a process that reduces analgesic availability before the drug enters the systemic circulation. Thus, higher oral dosages are required than via the parenteral route. See equianalgesic chart in Chapter 4.

Treat Procedural Pain Prophylactically

Procedural pain, while short-lived, deserves the same attention as any other acute pain experience. When approaching the problem, it is essential to address with the patient and/or family the expected intensity and duration of pain and anxiety secondary to the procedure. When procedures are ordered for diagnostic purposes, there may be significant meaning pertaining to the outcome that can result in even greater anxiety than that produced by anticipation of the pain alone.

Treat the painful procedure as a significant event. Prepare the patient for the procedure. An explanation detailing the steps in the procedure, the expected sensations, and the measures that will be taken to control discomfort can go a long way in calming the anxious patient. Diagrams or other visual aids may help. When anxiety cannot be controlled by cognitive intervention alone, it may be necessary to provide an anxiolytic agent or sedative in preparation for the procedure. Before beginning the procedure, also ensure that the patient's existing pain, if any, is well controlled.

Inasmuch as possible, perform the procedure on schedule to minimize anticipatory pain and anxiety. For procedures that are to be repeated, it is important to make the first experience as comfortable as possible to decrease subsequent fear. Assess the surroundings, privacy, patient and family needs, room temperature, and the presence of ominous-looking equipment.

Use nonpharmacologic measures to reduce pain. Tailor pain-relieving interventions to the patient's and the family's needs and preferences as well as the requirements of the procedure itself. Children may be comforted by the presence of a parent, and adults may also prefer significant others to remain in the room. The patient's preference should be honored if possible.

Parents may be asked to help their child through the procedure but should not be asked to restrain the child. Infants can benefit from touching and patting, and patients of all ages may benefit from the distraction that music provides.

Employ effective pharmacologic strategies. Administer medications as painlessly as possible. The oral and intravenous routes are far less traumatic than intramuscular injections. Local anesthetics, opioids, benzodiazepines, and/or barbiturates may be used. Local anesthetics are administered by infiltration or topical application. Opioids can be given orally or intravenously. The intravenous route provides the most rapid onset of action and allows for ease in titration until the desired analgesic effect is obtained. Benzodiazepines may be administered via multiple routes. They reduce anxiety and relax skeletal muscle but do not provide analgesia. Barbiturates also sedate without any direct analgesic effect, but have the disadvantage of having a long-lasting effect. Regardless of the agents chosen, the pharmacologic goal is to ensure that the patient can comfortably tolerate the procedure. Patients who are concurrently on opioid analgesic therapy or who have a chronic nonmalignant pain syndrome will require more analgesic than those who are opioid-naive.

Provide for Pain Relief across the Continuum of Care

The demands of the current health care delivery setting mandate earlier discharge from the acute care setting. These earlier discharges require increased vigilance to ensure that patients are adequately prepared to manage their pain on an outpatient basis. Predischarge assessment becomes of critical importance to prevent inadequately managed pain and/or a return to the acute care setting, often through the emergency department.

Assess analgesic requirements 24 hours before discharge. The patient's cumulative 24-hour analgesic dosage requirement allows for informed decision making when planning discharge medications. When assessing the patient's needs, it is important to take into consideration both scheduled and breakthrough analgesic dosing as well as any adjuvant medications that augment pain relief.

Provide discharge analgesics that are adequate and appropriate for outpatient use. Equianalgesic tables provide the data necessary for converting a parenteral analgesic to an oral one (see Chapter 4). Numerous oral analgesics are formulated as opioids alone or opioid-nonopioid compounds. For example, a postoperative patient has been receiving morphine 5 mg intravenously about every 6 hours. She is to be discharged the next morning. Vicodin 1 tablet is equianalgesic to 3 mg of parenteral morphine. She can be trialed on Vicodin 2 tablets every 4 to 6 hours prn for pain, no more than 8 in 24 hours. She could also be trialed on Percocet with one tablet equianalgesic to 2.4 mg parenteral morphine. Orders would read: Percocet 2 tablets every 4 to 6 hours, no more than 12 in 24 hours. If analgesic needs cannot be met because of the dose-limiting toxicity of the nonopioid in the compound, propoxyphene, oxycodone, morphine, and hydromorphone come in noncompounded formulations. It would be equally important to ensure that all medications necessary for pain relief are on hand. For example, an antispasmodic might be an essential part of the analgesic regimen. For patients who are not able to swallow well or not able to swallow at all, analgesic preparations are available in rectal formulations.

ROLE AND RESPONSIBILITY OF THE NURSE

Nursing's critical role in the management of acute pain is predicated on the fact that the nurse spends more time than any other health care professional in the presence of the person with pain. Given that the majority of acute pain treatment has a pharmacologic focus, the nurse's ability to ensure adequate management requires skilled assessment, intervention, and advocacy skills. Evaluation of treatment results based on a sound knowledge base of appropriate dosage, duration of effect, and side effect management positions the nurse to serve the patient well and effectively collaborate with other members of the health care team.

CASE STUDY

Joe, a 40-year-old male construction worker, is injured at work, sustaining a broken femur. He is admitted for surgery to repair the break and subsequently placed on a surgical unit. When he arrives on the surgical floor from the recovery room, he is moaning in pain and reports the pain intensity to be a 10 on a scale of 0 to 10. His face is contorted, his pulse at 110, and respiratory rate at 20. Transferring him to the hospital bed from the gurney produces a loud holler and much complaining. The nurse administers 10 mg of morphine intramuscularly. In about 40 minutes Joe reports a pain intensity of 6 on the same rating scale. The staff nurse calls the physician and asks for a change in analgesic orders. She requests discontinuance of the intramuscular route, utilization of an intravenous route, and a further loading dose of morphine at 2 mg every 10 minutes until the patient reports comfort or is drowsy. She further requests a scheduled dose of morphine 10 mg intravenously every four hours with dosage titration parameters. Parameters include: (1) increasing the scheduled dosage by 2 mg if relief does not last the full 4 hours and is reported to be more than 4 on a scale of 0 to 10 before the next scheduled dose; and (2) increasing the scheduled dosage by 4 mg if relief does not last the full 4 hours and is reported to be more than 6 on a scale of 0 to 10 before the next scheduled dose.

After the administration of 6 more milligrams of morphine as a loading dose, Joe evaluated the pain's intensity at a 3 (0–10 scale), a tolerable level for him. He required an increase in the scheduled dosage to 12 mg and was then comfortable for the following 36 hours. His analgesic needs were converted to an equianalgesic oral dose when his pain level dropped to less than 5 and he was able to tolerate oral intake.

Clinical Accountabilities

1. Assess adequately and frequently.
   - Have the patient rate the pain level before and after the analgesic is administered. Consistently use the same rating scale after ensuring the patient understands its structure.
   - Ensure that pain relief is adequate until the next analgesic dose can be given.
   - Determine whether any activities exacerbate pain intensity.
   - Monitor for analgesic side effects.

2. Deal appropriately with the patient when relief is inadequate.
   - Don't tell the patient that the analgesic should have worked, that he must endure the pain, or that nothing else can be done.
   - Do assure the patient that you will communicate with the physician for a change in orders and will maximize the use of existing ordered analgesics.

3. Effectively communicate the patient's status to the physician and other health team members in a timely manner.
   - Provide an articulate and concise pain assessment based on the patient's self-report.
   - Include location, intensity, and specific sensations.
   - Describe the response to ordered analgesics: the drug, dosage, route, duration of relief, and side effects.

4. Have a sound pharmacologic knowledge base.
   - Understand equianalgesic conversion.
   - Know the efficacy of varied routes.
   - Be familiar with the expected duration of effect of the various analgesics.

5. Advocate for the patient.
   - Request treatment changes when relief is inadequate.

Continued on following page

Clinical Accountabilities *(Continued)*

— Articulate when a particular drug/dosage has been maximized. Make suggestions for specific changes, such as drug, route, dosage, schedule.
— Refer to reference/research articles as appropriate.
— Address bias/misconceptions from other members of the health care team.

6. Assist the patient/family to be knowledgeable consumers and effective advocates.
   — Prepare the preoperative patient for location and type of pain, kind of assessment tool utilized, and expected management plan.
   — Provide instruction on the importance of preventative intervention, such as stopping the pain before it starts.
   — If medication is available only on an as-needed basis, instruct the patient to ask for the analgesic when pain starts.

7. Maximize the existing treatment regimen.
   — Administer analgesics ordered on an as-needed basis on schedule if the pain is consistent or expected to be consistent.
   — If more than one drug or route is ordered, choose the most effective one for the patient's situation.
   — If there are dosage or titration parameters, use those orders effectively.
   — Promptly treat any analgesic side effects.

8. Document the patient's status and response to analgesic interventions.
   — Drug, dosage, and route administered.
   — Pain level before and after administration.
   — Efficacy of nonpharmacologic interventions.

BIBLIOGRAPHY

Acute Pain Management Guideline Panel. (1992). *Acute pain management: Operative or medical procedures and trauma. Clinical practice guideline.* AHCPR Pub. No. 92-0032. Rockville, MD.: Agency for Health Care Policy and Research, Public Health Service, U.S. Department of Health and Human Services.

American Pain Society. (1992). *Principles of analgesic use in the treatment of acute pain and cancer pain* (3rd ed.). Skokie, IL.: American Pain Society.

Bonica, J.J. (1990). General considerations of acute pain. In J.J. Bonica (Ed.), *The management of pain* (2nd ed., pp. 159–179). Philadelphia: Lea & Febiger.

McCaffery, M., & Beebe, A. (1989). Pharmacological control of pain: A multidisciplinary approach. In M. McCaffery & A. Beebe (Eds.), *Pain. Clinical manual for nursing practice* (pp. 42–123). St. Louis: Mosby.

Rapp, S.E., Ready, L.B., & Nessly, M.L. (1995). Acute pain management in patients with prior opioid consumption: A case-controlled retrospective review. *Pain 61*(2), 195–201.

Warfield, C.A., & Kahn, C.H. (1995). Acute pain management. Programs in U.S. hospitals and experiences and attitudes among U.S. adults. *Anesthesiology 83*(5), 1090–1094.

9
Chronic Nonmalignant Pain

As Bonica said, **chronic pain** is "pain that persists a month beyond the usual course of an acute disease or a reasonable time for an injury to heal or that is associated with a chronic pathologic process that causes continuous pain or the pain recurs at intervals for months or years" (1990, p. 19), and nonmalignant pain is associated with conditions other than cancer.

Chronic nonmalignant pain is not simply an extension of acute pain for a prolonged time. It is in itself a complex disease state that may seriously affect quality of life (Bonica, 1990). Millions of people experience chronic nonmalignant pain each year with varying degrees of disability secondary to unrelieved pain. Although acute pain may serve as a warning or protective mechanism, chronic pain has no such value. On the contrary, chronic pain drains the individual and affects every aspect of his or her life. To provide effective care, the health care worker must first recognize the significant differences between acute and chronic pain (Table 9–1).

MULTIDIMENSIONALITY

Chronic pain is more complex than acute pain. Relief of chronic pain cannot be effectively achieved without thoroughly addressing physiologic, emotional, social, and economic aspects. These other facets potentiate the pain and increase the patient's vulnerability in a way that weaves a complicated clinical challenge. Lack of concentration, sleeplessness, over- or undereating, diminished activity, role disruption, social isolation, altered self-image, job loss, financial insecurity, and an endless search for relief are some of the elements that

TABLE 9–1   *Differences Between Acute Pain and Chronic Pain*

Acute Pain	Chronic Pain
Precipitating event with evidence of tissue damage	May have no identifiable pathophysiology
Well-defined pattern of onset	Often irregular, ill-defined pattern of onset
Normal defense mechanism that brings attention to underlying problem	No useful purpose as a warning mechanism
Common physiologic responses: elevated pulse and blood pressure, diaphoresis	Physiologic adaptation with normalization of pulse and blood pressure
Serotonin and endorphin levels usually increased	Serotonin and endorphin levels often decreased, lowering pain threshold
Resolution of pain with restoration of normal tissue function: short-term and self-limited	Lasts months to years and persists despite healing or resolution of original cause
Usually responsive to standard interventions	Response to standard interventions elusive: multiple interventions usually needed

permeate the patient's life. Often the pain experience becomes all-encompassing and dominates the person's entire existence. Although individuals vary in their response to pain, the clinician must be sensitive and responsive to the multidimensionality of chronic pain.

Fear, Worry, and Sleep Disturbances

Sleep disturbances due to the pain itself and to fear and worry are common. It may be difficult to find a position that offers adequate comfort to promote sleep. Yet, lying quietly, free of distractions, may not actually be conducive to sleep. On the contrary, a mind not diverted with other thoughts may focus on the illness, pain, and other stressful issues. Often, patients are concerned about the cause of their pain, wondering whether there is something more seriously wrong than they have been told. They worry, too, that there will be no end to the pain or that the pain will become even worse. When the patient has been unable to work, economic concerns may interfere with sleep. Whether caused by pain or anxiety, sleep deprivation is a frequent partner of chronic pain, leaving patients tired and irritable and hypersensitive to pain and to other stimuli.

Lack of Concentration/Irritability

Hypersensitivity to Pain

Constant pain and inadequate sleep deplete defenses and further lower pain tolerance, causing a response that is totally out of proportion for a minimal injury. Such excessive responses may be perceived to be overreaction and/or manipulation; however, the patient experiences the "minor pain" intensely. Lack of concentration and irritability also occur. Inability to concentrate interferes with the patient's performance at work or home and decreases self-confidence. Irritability alienates others with one of two typical outcomes. Either people avoid the patient because of the irritability or (if the patient is cognizant of the irritable behavior) she or he avoids others to prevent negative interactions from occurring. In either event, avoidance promotes social isolation.

Physical Limitations

Pain dictates physical activity and activities are consciously or unconsciously limited to avoid additional discomfort. Compensatory mechanisms (e.g., unnatural position of any body part to avoid exacerbating pain) contribute to limitations beyond the original pathologic process. Sheer physical exhaustion also reduces activity. Patients are severely drained of energy from sleeplessness and efforts to cope with the pain and to conceal it from others. A combination of diminished physical activity and unpredictable pain patterns reinforces social isolation.

Role Changes

It is not unusual for social roles to change. For example, a father may assume maternal tasks to help an incapacitated mother, a wife may become the breadwinner when the husband is no longer able to work, a child may take on parental responsibilities to fill a void. Although role flexibility can be enriching in some situations, the permanency of the pain and subsequent demands can be overwhelming for family members and depressing for the patient. The patient and family experience an invasion of their social beings.

Gastrointestinal Implications

Eating habits change. Some patients experience loss of appetite with subsequent loss of weight. Conversely, others are restless and eat compulsively. In the latter case, the overeating and reduced physical activity combine to cause excessive weight gain. Either extreme has a negative impact on the already challenged self-image. Constipation is a common problem, caused by improper eating, inadequate exercise, and medication side effects.

Financial Losses

These various dimensions of chronic pain take an economic toll as well. Patients may never be able to return to their original job, leaving them and their families with serious financial problems. Those who do return to work may have reduced hours or a lower-paying job to accommodate their restrictions. This, too, can create financial concerns. Even those who resume their original work fear economic loss. These patients often increase their own stress by trying to conceal their pain and its personal implications. In addition to direct economic loss, there is the financial loss incurred by the vigilant search for the magic medication that will finally relieve the pain. Desperate for help, patients often try any medications, any treatments at any cost in their endless search. This adds financial burden to a patient and family already strained by the other aspects of chronic pain.

Living with pain is stressful in itself and the patient becomes increasingly more vulnerable as one or all of the above elements are extensions of and integral parts of the entire pain experience. Chronic pain is like a pebble thrown into a pond: There is a distinctive dip where the stone breaks the surface surrounded by many concentric circles, none of which can be separated from the entire stone-throwing episode.

OCCURRENCE

According to the American Pain Society, 45% of all Americans experience persistent pain for which they need help at some time in their lives. Headache and low-back pain are the most common of the "intractable" or difficult-to-relieve pains reported. To demonstrate the magnitude of the problem, it is helpful to note that 150 million workdays are lost every year because of headache alone! Yet, there are multiple conditions that produce chronic pain. The following examples, though not an exhaustive list, may serve to emphasize the extent of chronic pain in our society:

- Amputation (phantom pain, stump pain)
- Ankylosing spondylitis
- Arthritis, rheumatoid, and osteoarthritis
- Causalgia
- Crohn's disease
- Chronic pancreatitis
- Diabetic peripheral neuropathy
- Fibrositis
- Guillain-Barré neuropathy
- Headache (migraine, cluster, tension, vascular, etc.)
- Hemophilia (with bleeding into closed spaces)
- Irritable bowel syndrome
- Low-back pain
- Neck pain (such as whiplash)
- Trigeminal or postherpetic neuralgia
- Vascular diseases of limbs (e.g., Raynaud's disease)
- Reflex sympathetic dystrophy
- Sickle cell disease

COMPLEXITY OF ASSESSMENT

Chronic pain cannot be assessed or treated in a simplistic way. Although pain instruments may be used for both chronic and acute pain, they must be part of a much more extensive assessment. Ideally, all patient care is holistic; relief of chronic pain, in particular, must be holistic or fail.

Physiologically, acute and chronic pain differ. Persistent chronic pain eventually produces change in the patient's natural response to pain. For example, chronic pain reduces serotonin and endorphin levels, lowering the pain threshold. Thus the patient's pain may be more intense than if it had been caused by an acute phenomenon. This is contrary to the perceptions most health care workers hold, and therefore it is important for the clinician to understand prolonged pain effects to ensure adequate assessment and intervention.

The irony of chronic pain is that chronicity itself reduces evidence of pain. The body compensates to normalize pulse, blood pressure, and other autonomic responses, eliminating these as corroborative data. The clinician familiar with acute pain assessment may misinterpret the normal vital signs as an absence of or lessened pain. Facial expressions and body signs associated with pain, also may not be dependable for chronic pain assessment. Sheer fatigue may dull expression, although the pain persists. To conceal pain and disability patients often modify behaviors to mask the presence of pain. For example, grimacing and guarding are typical manifestations of acute pain, yet these may be entirely absent in patients who have learned to control their response to constant pain. When such adaptations have occurred, the clinician will not find physical signs to support the patient's complaint of pain.

Often, this leaves the patient's description as the primary determinant of the pain experience. This is difficult for clinicians who are educated to gather a variety of indications to build a clinical picture. Test results and other substantiation of the underlying condition may be of assistance; however, it is essential to understand that with chronic pain there may be no other evidence than the patient's statement to form the basis of pain intervention (e.g., low-back pain, migraine headaches, phantom pain). The fundamental precept that must be remembered is that the patient is the only authority about his or her pain (McCaffery & Beebe, 1989).

Having said that, there is one warning about the patient account of chronic pain. The clinician must be aware that sometimes patients understate their pain in an effort to please the family or health care professionals. Fear of rejection or desire to avoid "being a burden" may result in the patient's downplaying the pain they are experiencing. This behavior should be considered with any patient, but particularly the elderly (see Chapter 12). Developing trust and being nonjudgmental are critical to open, honest communication with such patients.

Despite the limitations described, there are no absolute generalities when treating chronic pain. Each person must have an all-inclusive, objective evaluation to determine individual response. The dimensions mentioned in this chapter also must be weighed to ensure that functionality and quality of life are considered in the overall assessment. The practitioner may use any one of several assessment tools to gather information about the pain experience.

GUIDELINES FOR COMPREHENSIVE CHRONIC PAIN ASSESSMENT

Physical Observations

What is the degree of mobility for activities of daily living (ADLs), such as feeding, bathing/hygiene, toileting, dressing, and generalized movements?

Are movements or activities avoided? If so, what are they?

What compensating positions or movements are employed?

Are autonomic responses present: elevated blood pressure, increased pulse and respiration, dilated pupils, diaphoresis? *Note: These may not be evident in chronic pain, as discussed.*

What effects do medications, treatments, or other variants have on mobility and complaint of pain?

What do test results show about the type and degree of underlying pathology?

KEY POINT

Amount of pathology and degree of pain are not necessarily proportional.

What is the length and pattern of sleep?

Is constipation a problem? Consider medications, activity, and eating habits.

Does patient appear fatigued, drained, lifeless?

Pain History (obtain from patient and family)

When did the pain begin initially?

Was onset sudden (e.g., after an injury) or gradual?

What activities or events trigger or elevate pain levels?

What helps to relieve pain?

What medications are taken for pain? What medications have been used unsuccessfully for pain relief? What medications are taken for reasons other than pain? Consider interactions and side effects of medications.

What treatments/procedures have been tried? What worked well?

Role Appraisal

What tasks are done in the home, such as cooking, shopping, driving, or small repairs. Are these different from before?

Has there been a shift in roles within the family? Such role changes might include a child taking on parental responsibilities for siblings, providing care to the patient, doing work usually done by one of the parents. Or these changes may be the partner becoming the breadwinner for the first time, assuming tasks in the household previously done by the patient. The marital relationship may no longer be an equal partnership.

Did the patient have employment when the pain started, and if so, is she or he still employed?

If employed, is the job the same?

If the job is not the same, what was the nature of the change?

Is the patient off work frequently. If so, how often/ long?

Has there been significant financial effect of changed or lost work? Litigation?

Self-Esteem/Social Evaluation

Is the patient irritable or short-tempered with others?

Does the patient often appear tired or withdrawn from conversation and activities?

Have social activities been progressively reduced? Be specific, such as going to movies or ballgames, attending church, having or going to parties.

Have family members experienced a reduction of social activities?

How do the patient and family get along? Is there anger, avoidance, guilt, and/or other emotion that needs attention?

Does the entire family appear functional or dysfunctional in their interactions?

Patient Account

What does the pain feel like? Do not lead the patient, but note his or her words, such as dull, throbbing, gnawing.

How would you rate your pain? Use any standard assessment scale to obtain rating, and consistently use the same scale.

Is the pain constant, or does it come and go?

If it is intermittent, what makes it start or stop?

How extensive is the pain, that is, how large an area does the pain involve? *It has been found that there is a relationship between the extent of pain and report of duration (Krause, Tiat, & Margolis, 1989).*

What do you do to cope with the pain?

To what extent do you feel the pain has affected your life?

Do you ever feel depressed? Have you ever felt so overwhelmed that you wanted to die?

KEY POINT

It is important to recognize that depression does not cause pain, but unrelieved pain can cause depression.

Throughout the entire assessment, the clinician must remain open and nonjudgmental. The patient must feel that she or he is respected and believed to freely discuss this most personal experience, pain, without fear of rejection or need to conform to "expected" behavior. This sounds like a simple matter. However, many factors can obstruct the relationship and ultimately the road to pain relief. To manage pain effectively, the clinician must first recognize and then act to reduce or eliminate barriers.

BARRIERS TO PAIN RELIEF

Factors that have a negative impact on pain relief in general have been discussed previously in Chapter 8, Acute Pain. It should be noted that, in addition, there are barriers specific to chronic pain management that need to be identified and confronted by the health care practitioner.

Disconnectedness

As mentioned in this chapter, severity of chronic pain can be as great or greater than that of acute pain. Yet, societal and even health care perceptions of chronic pain are that it is somehow less intense than acute pain, perhaps because acute pain is most often accompanied with some visible evidence of the traumatic cause, providing an emotional reality for the observer, an experience they can personalize and "feel." For example, postoperative pain is understood in the context of a surgical incision, burn pain through the damaged skin, trauma pain through wounds, and so on. Perhaps chronic pain, lacking such dramatic links, fails to translate.

Clinician Bias

The gnarled hands of the arthritic patient are certainly tangible evidence of a pathologic process. Yet, the discomfort and lifestyle impact of this chronic condition often are greatly underestimated. Clinicians have difficulty relating to the experience. Why? What explains greater or lesser empathy in different situations? Strauss and Glaser (1975) noted that reactions to the visible signs of chronic illness were "not simply a matter of physiological appearance but of learned perceptual capacities." This would explain variability of clinician response when physical evidence supports the patient's complaint of pain. Clinicians not only assess, but also tend to interpret pain. And those interpretations are skewed by their own life experiences and beliefs, particularly in a society and profession that view disease in an acute model.

Most health care practitioners have had little formal preparation for managing pain, let alone the challenges of chronic pain. They come to the clinical situation with a variety of beliefs, both their long-standing personal ones and those they have acquired in health care settings. Physicians tend to be conservative and underprescribe, selecting less potent drugs, lower-than-needed dosages, and longer intervals between doses. Nurses often unconsciously reduce effectiveness further by using the lowest dosage ordered at the least frequent intervals. This ineffectual approach to pain management is typical of both acute and chronic situations. The difference in chronic pain is that the situation is exacerbated by the concern of addiction over time or the suspicion that the patient is really a substance abuser who is manipulating to obtain more medications. Indeed, the behavior of the chronic pain patient may reinforce these assumptions. Failure to exhibit the classical picture of pain is a major impediment for most health care professionals to accurately assess and treat pain.

For decades, health care has been based on a disease/acute model, that is, focused on saving lives in crisis and on curing illness. It is very difficult for health care professionals in such a model to accept the fact that they may not be able to save all lives, cure all diseases, or relieve all pain and suffering. The entire focus is to "win" against the challenges, whatever those may be. Caring for patients with persistent pain that defies interventions creates a feeling of "failure" for the practitioner. They cannot beat this formidable opponent called chronic pain. Without realizing they are doing so, practitioners may begin to avoid these patients, not wishing to be reminded of their own perceived inadequacy. Or, practitioners unfamiliar with chronic pain may perceive behavior that does not conform to expectation as manipulation. The very patients who need them most become even more isolated with their problem.

CASE STUDY

Consider Jennie, aged 29, who interacts little with anyone except to request pain medication (75 mg Demerol q 4 hr PRN) for her low-back pain. In an effort to deal with her pain, Jennie reads one novel after another for distraction. She remains immersed in a story for long periods without any outward evidence of pain, yet watches the clock for her medication and becomes upset if the medication is "late." Her physician and nurses, who are unfamiliar with chronic pain, are not able to identify the real issue. They cannot see the situation as one of unrelieved pain, so they begin to think Jennie is faking the pain to obtain medication for mood alteration. They become angry at being manipulated, and a cycle of lost trust begins. Feeling she is not believed, Jennie becomes more anxious, has more pain, and tries to gain greater control of her medication. This behavior further alienates the health care practitioners until an adversarial relationship is perpetuated. Sadly, Jennie, so harshly judged, was simply trying to cope with her pain. Practitioners skillful with chronic pain management would have supported her coping strategies, evaluated alternative medications and dosing, and explored with Jennie other options for pain relief. Rather than a manipulative scenario, this is a typical example of unrelieved pain and the patient's effort to "get through" another day of pain.

Although pain knows no age restrictions, the elderly frequently are affected with chronic pain (see Chapter 12). In a society that values youth, immediate responses (consider E-mail, faxes, and interactive computers), and productivity through employment, the elderly patient with chronic pain requires a different mind-set and approach from the norm. Patience (especially with the slower pace that may be required for some elderly patients), effective listening skills, and sensitivity to the special needs of the older adult are necessary. Chronic pain is not less important than acute pain or disease management itself. Respect for the patient's pain experience is at the heart of seeking a resolution to the problem. It is imperative that clinicians not view arthritic and other chronic, painful disorders as part of the aging process and, thus, as necessary evils that must be endured.

Fear of Addiction

Fear of addiction may prevail in any pain situation, but chronic pain situations are thought by many to be fraught with this danger because of the lack of time limitations. Opioids have been administered lightly or not at all for chronic pain because of this inaccurate information. Withholding opioids often has meant withholding adequate pain relief to sufferers. Contrary to common belief, opioids (the word "narcotics" is deliberately not used here to avoid possible association with street drugs) do not usually cause addiction when taken for pain. Although tolerance may develop over time, it must be remembered that this is not the same as addiction. Patients using opioids for pain relief experience improved function and are able to control use. This is in contrast to people with substance use disorders who use opioids for mood alteration and cannot control use (see Chapter 13). Opioids are not the first choice for chronic pain, but, when managed appropriately, they can provide effective, safe pain relief for intractable pain.

Communication Problems

Language difficulties or cultural beliefs that inhibit open communications may be present in chronic or acute pain situations. In addition, the subtleties of long-standing chronic pain may create other communication barriers. For example, verbal and physical communication of pain is diminished with long-term chronic pain. Patients may not admit to pain to please the health care professional or avoid rejection. They may deny the pain to avoid injections or treatments or fail to respond from fear of addiction or loss of control. Elderly patients, fearing loss of independence, may understate discomfort. At the other extreme, patients who have had secondary gain from the sick role may unconsciously cling to their present situation, exaggerating their disability. Perhaps least understood are the patients who have had repeated treatment failures and who are very demanding about pain relief. These patients are fearful of another failure—failure to obtain relief or even convince others of their suffering. Although their behavior is the cry of desperation, it often results in rejection because it does not conform to acceptable behavior. Relentless pain and decreased quality of life can result in depression that often is perceived as the cause rather than the result of the pain experience. Such patients are grossly misunderstood. They are perceived to be imagining their pain instead of defeated by the constancy of suffering. The chronicity of the pain experience and quality of life concerns will precipitate a number of different responses that must be recognized and incorporated into the plan of care.

In any event, the patient with chronic pain is likely to have more difficulty making the pain experience understood by clinicians or family alike than their counterpart with acute pain. Even when the pain is accepted, clinician beliefs may contribute to less than adequate pain intervention. Clinicians must consider and work through their own and others' beliefs regarding chronic pain so that they do not deny patients their due rights to appropriate care.

PATIENT CARE MEASURES

Building Trust

It is essential to build trust with the patient. Listening is the first step, not just hearing, but accepting whatever the patient says about the pain without judgment. Acknowledging the existence and intensity of pain as described by the patient will, in itself, reduce his or her stress and fear of unrelieved pain. If the patient has been unexpressive, the mere gesture of honest concern may, in time, be enough to release those suppressed feelings. Accepting the pain also means accepting the patient.

A significant responsibility in chronic pain management is to alleviate the fear of pain, which exists between the most intense pain periods. The relentless cycle of chronic pain provides no respite, no time of full comfort (Figure 9–1).

Demonstrating sincere interest in and acceptance of the pain is the first step in breaking the cycle of fear

FIGURE 9–1   *The Circle of Chronic Pain*

and pain. Trust is established when the patient believes the health care professional understands and is responsive to his or her pain experience. To put it simply, relationships are everything.

Establish Ownership

Chronic pain is complicated, and complete relief may not be a realistic goal. The health care practitioner must beware of falling back into the acute model and expecting to "cure" the pain. By definition, chronic pain persists and recurs over time. Depending on the underlying cause, the pain may continue for life, requiring a variety of strategies to minimize discomfort and disability. It may not be possible to fully eliminate it.

Initially, the patient and clinician form a partnership in accepting and resolving chronic pain, a commitment that extends to the entire health care team. As effective pain management evolves, the patient role should become more active, one of owning the pain and its relief. A fundamental rule for the clinician is to empower the patient to manage his or her own pain. The clinician must not be a rescuer, but rather a partner and facilitator for the patient to take charge of the pain and ultimately his or her own life. As appropriate strategies are identified and implemented, the patient should become more and more secure, feel greater control of the pain and its relief. Success should be measured by the ability of the patient to minimize pain and maintain a relatively normal existence. Realistic goals of chronic pain management would be (1) to minimize pain; (2) to maximize functional capacity; and (3) to help the patient recognize his or her own power over the pain experience. Without patient ownership, real help is only temporary.

Involve the Family

Although pain is a personal experience, it is not limited to the person in whom it originates. Pain is a human and social experience as well as a physiologic and emotional one. The person experiencing chronic pain must live with the pain, as will their family and others close to the individual. The family knows the pain as it affects their relationship with the loved one and its impact on their own lives. Their compassion for the suffering of their loved one often is understandably mixed with anger and resentment for the changes it imposes on their freedom. Even the greatest love is tested mightily by the length and endurance of this burden. However, martyrdom is not beneficial, either. Those who silently succumb to all demands may appear the most supportive, yet may be contributing to a dependent role and downward spiral for the patient. There is no "perfect" family response, only that which is most manageable and the least invasive to the lives of all concerned.

Simply observing the interaction with family members will give the clinician additional information about how effectively the family is managing the pain experience. The clinician should be keenly aware of the social interactions and roles each individual family member is assuming. Not only spoken words and overt actions, but also the words and actions withheld should be noted.

CASE STUDY

Sarah, 80 years old, suffers from osteoarthritis. She lives with her sister, Dorothy, aged 76. Her younger sister is very solicitous of Sarah's needs, waiting on her extensively. This has developed into a situation in which Sarah plays a dependent, sick role and seeks pain relief and gratification through the interventions of others, predominately Dorothy. As pointed out, effective pain management is anchored in patients' ownership of their own experience. Sarah is caught in a cycle of passivity and inadequate pain relief that results in increased demands. From the perspective of her caregiver sister, Dorothy, the responsibility that was assumed readily at first has now become a burden. As Sarah's demands increase, her sister tires more easily because of her own age and health and the endless efforts she must expend. Dorothy begins to feel victimized and trapped by Sarah's illness. Although well-intentioned, the coping style of this family cannot achieve effective pain management and is negatively affecting the lives of both parties. The clinician, assessing the nontherapeutic relationship, would direct interventions toward establishing ownership and creating a healthier interaction between the two sisters. It is obvious that this cannot be done with the patient alone; both members of the family will need to understand fully the gains that are possible and how to accomplish them.

The family cannot be separated from the pain management process. The clinician, considering the patient as part of the family unit, will involve family members in each step of the process: assessment, planning, intervention, and evaluation. A family member may give valuable information that the patient failed to mention or give insight into some of the responses given that will assist in a valid assessment. Because chronic pain has so many dimensions that affect the entire family, it is critical that the family understand and support the pain management plan that is developed. Although the patient must assume responsibility for pain relief, this does not imply that she or he can do so in isolation. Family members can reinforce desired behaviors and provide support in changing lifestyle. Conversely, if excluded, family may inadvertently encourage old behaviors and contribute to the patient reverting to ineffective responses.

CASE STUDY

At age 34 Carolyn suffers from sciatica. She states that pain is less bearable in the late afternoon, but can offer no explanation for this. Her husband, on the other hand, points out that after school their children have friends over to play and that the patient insists on preparing the dinner. These activities that are not, in themselves, unusual can contribute to activity that is excessive. A plan that might help set a more constructive pace could be alternating the play location, one day at Carolyn's home and the next at a neighbor's home. On the afternoon the children play elsewhere Carolyn could cook, thereby fulfilling her need to demonstrate her homemaker role while not exceeding her capacity. Or perhaps a baby-sitter could be arranged (a teenager seeking income, a church volunteer, or a friend) for a short period to ensure further rest. Perhaps meal planning could include use of a crockpot or cooking in volume and freezing foods for the weekdays. These are just some possible ways to keep Carolyn's valued activities without exceeding her physical capacity. Her husband's input offered important insight into the reality of Carolyn's home situation. The point is twofold: (1) even the smallest bit of information helps put the home environment in perspective; and (2) to be effective, pain management must address the patient's life as it exists and has meaning to the individual. Creativity mixed with pain management principles will forge a viable plan for the patient and family.

Include the Whole Health Care Team

The multifaceted nature of chronic pain demands a multidisciplinary approach for effective resolution. Various members of the health care team collaborate to provide required therapies for pain relief and/or improved function. Nurses, pharmacists, dietitians, physical therapists, and other specialized personnel work in concert with the physician to achieve pain management goals. Social services can be invaluable in assessing and making recommendations related to the financial and social problems that can undermine even the best program. Every member of the health care team, regardless of his or her position, must fully understand the plan for the patient and be accountable for supporting designated behaviors. This includes not only all disciplines, but also those within each discipline who interact with the patient (such as technical dand assistive personnel). For example, the nursing assistant who helps the patient with ADLs must know the patient's capabilities, limits, and how specifically to contribute toward positive behaviors. Good communication with each team member will ensure consistent responses to both the patient and family and facilitate progress.

Employ a Multimodal Approach

In contrast to acute pain management, which is predominately based on a pharmacologic approach, the foundation of chronic pain management is nonpharmacologic, with medications adjunctive rather than primary components of relief. Although analgesics have a place in the treatment of chronic pain, it is important to realize that therapy is patient centered. Cognitive strategies are employed to shift the patient from victim to controller by changing pain perceptions and responses. The patient learns to pace activities and eliminate or reduce stressors. From that starting point, numerous nonpharmacologic interventions and some pharmacologic supplements can be beneficial.

Although treatment modalities vary somewhat depending on the underlying disorder, the commonality is that multiple interventions are the norm for persistent pain. Neither chronic pain nor its relief are simple. Several treatment modalities are usually combined to accomplish adequate relief. Chronic pain therapy may be compared more easily to treatment of other complex disorders or diseases than to acute pain management, which generally is responsive to analgesics. For example, diabetes mellitus is not simply regulating blood sugar with insulin; therapy includes diet, smoking cessation, physical activity, foot care, eye exams, and all aspects that relate to the central disease. Similarly, chronic pain management requires a comprehensive regimen. Therapy is commensurate with its innate complexity and tailored to meet the individual's needs.

Nonpharmacologic interventions include both cognitive-behavioral and physical agents. Foremost among cognitive-behavioral approaches is education. It is through education that patients can understand and learn to cope with their pain. With their commitment and participation, relaxation and distraction techniques, imagery, biofeedback, and music therapy may be used. Yoga, meditation, and other stress-reducing activities may be chosen; skilled practitioners may assist with hypnosis in select cases. Cognitive strategies are frequently employed as part of the management of chronic pain because they improve quality of life and promote the patient's sense of control.

Physical agents encompass a wide assortment of pain relief measures. Chronic muscle and joint discomfort often is relieved by moist or dry heat. Superficial measures include heating pads, hot packs, hot baths, saunas, and whirlpools. Diathermy, and more commonly ultrasound, provide methods of deep heat application to joints and other sites. Although chronic pain due to muscle, joint, or soft-tissue pathology is responsive to heat, neurologically induced pain may be more effectively treated with cold. In addition to cold packs applied locally, cold may be applied to acupoints (acupuncture points) or directed at peripheral nerves via cryoprobes.

Massage is used to relieve pain by relaxing muscles and reducing muscle spasm. Superficial massage of the back has a twofold purpose, that of relieving tension and relaxing muscles. When deep massage is provided by a skilled practitioner, one or more deep muscles can be manipulated to relieve spasm. Physical therapy and exercise are essential for maintaining and improving function. As noted, patients in pain reduce their activity and assume unnatural positions to avoid additional pain. Such responses further decrease their physical functioning level and contribute to increased pain when activity occurs. A basic principle of chronic pain management is to maximize functionality. Appropriate exercise and/or physical therapy are important to maximizing physical condition, but they also contribute to overall well-being by keeping the patient in the mainstream and preventing the isolation that can occur from progressive inactivity.

Transcutaneous electrical nerve stimulation (TENS) units may be effective in relieving chronic back pain, phantom limb pain, and pain due to radiculopathies and compression syndromes. Neurogenic pain (due to postherpetic or trigeminal neuralgia, peripheral nerve injury, etc.) may also respond to TENS. Patients differ greatly in their response to TENS, so it is wise to test effectiveness prior to purchasing such an expensive device. Under research is laser therapy in which pain-sensitive neurons are selectively destroyed. Potentially laser therapy could relieve intractable pain such as causalgia, phantom limb pain, and back pain (*Canadian Critical Care Nursing Journal,* 1990–91).

Alternatives to conventional therapy include those built on the energy field theory. Some of these are therapeutic touch, meridian tracing (light massage at points along specific pathways of the body), acupressure, and reflexology (massage of hands or feet to provide analgesia in corresponding zone) (Owens & Ehrenreich, 1991). Whether alternative interventions have or have not been scientifically supported, the fact is that they often produce effective pain relief. Clinicians must open their minds to new possibilities to assist those in whom conventional therapy has failed.

More invasive treatment may be appropriate, particularly when there is nerve involvement. Sympathetic blocks, IV administration of or subcutaneous infiltration with local anesthetics, and neurosurgical (often stereotaxical) surgical procedures are some options. Myofascial pain has successfully been treated by injections of local anesthetics at trigger points. Less invasive and less conventional is acupuncture, an ancient Chinese therapy that is getting more attention in Western medical circles.

Pharmacologic support is most commonly with nonopiates, such as salicylates or nonsteroidal anti-inflammatory drugs (NSAIDs). Acetaminophen may be used; however, because it has no anti-inflammatory effects, it is limited to disorders that do not require that action. Salicylates include aspirin, diflusinal, salsalate, and choline/magnesium salicylate. There are numerous NSAIDs, such as diclofenac, flurbiprofen, ibuprofen, tolmetin, and sulindac (for an extensive list and dosages, see Chapter 4). NSAIDs have properties similar to those of aspirin, but have greater potency (Malseed & Wilson, 1993). Although salicylates and NSAIDs often are successfully administered for chronic pain, such as rheumatoid and osteoarthritis pain, their untoward side effects should not be underestimated. In addition to the gastrointestinal irritation and decreased platelet aggregation shared by both salicylates and NSAIDs, NSAIDs also may cause drug-induced renal insufficiency and nephrotoxicity. Use in the elderly or those with preexisting medical conditions must be carefully evaluated.

Opioids, though not a first-line choice, may have a place in some situations of intractable pain not relieved by other medications and interventions. Contrary to widespread belief, rapid escalation of doses is not common in chronic opioid therapy in order to achieve pain relief (Portenoy, 1990). Small incremental increases in opioids spread over months or years may provide effective pain relief and improved function for some patients. It must be remembered that a substance is not the sole factor in potential addiction. In addition, "a variety of physiologic, psychologic and social factors . . . predispose the individual to this outcome" (Portenoy, 1990).

When opioid therapy is used, the goal is to achieve a regimen that provides pain relief without reinforcing dependency on the medication. As mentioned, central to chronic pain management is the concept that the patient must take responsibility for pain relief. Medications must be used to supplement, not drive, pain relief and to support the patient as the controller. Long-acting opioids, such as methadone or transdermal fentanyl (Duragesic®), may be among the choices because they remove the "focus" from taking an analgesic preparation. For identified patients with chronic nonmalignant pain who might benefit from opioid therapy and who are not opioid-naive (i.e., who have been taking chronic doses of an oral opioid preparation), the application of a Duragesic® patch every 3 days has some appeal. As with any analgesic preparation, monitoring and frequent reassessment are required. Epidural analgesia with opioids may be indicated (see Chapter 5).

Antidepressants may be needed, at least initially, to help the patient take charge of the pain situation. Unending pain, social, emotional and/or financial impacts may have so overwhelmed the patient that she or he cannot mobilize energy to get control. As mentioned, the clinician must understand that the depression is the result, not the cause, of the pain. Patients who have endured prolonged, unrelieved pain and its effects are so burdened that they cannot immediately help themselves.

Some interventions work especially well for certain disorders. These are not rigid regimens, but rather interventions that are particularly suited to the specific cause. For example, therapy for low-back pain may consist of sauna or whirlpool, strength training, and aerobic fitness. Muscle relaxants and/or analgesics may be appropriate supplements; however, the focus is on creating a healthier state. Sleep may be enhanced by proper positioning, relaxation or distraction techniques, or perhaps some well-selected music to raise the pain threshold at bedtime. Cognitive-behavioral elements are combined with physical agents and supplemented pharmacologically. Note that the patient plays an active role in managing pain. Follow-through depends on the patient, as does implementation of sleep-inducing techniques. The patient must apply the principles to achieve sustained relief.

It should be clear from the wide variety of interventions, both pharmacologic and nonpharmacologic, that there is no standard treatment(s) for chronic pain. The cause of pain will be a factor in selecting interventions, as will the patient's individual response. The clinician's role is to help the patient by introducing possibilities and identifying those that meet the needs of that individual. The one absolute in chronic pain management is that there must be a comprehensive, multimodal approach that places the patient in command.

CASE STUDY

Marian presented with postradiation fibrosis; diffuse scar tissue secondary to radiation was causing severe L4–S5 pain. Marian displayed considerable anxiety due to persistent, unrelieved pain despite multiple pain medications. Assessment revealed she had inordinate stress in her life. This is a fairly typical presentation of chronic pain effects, with the patient exhibiting either severe anxiety or, more frequently, depression as a result of intractable pain.

A benzodiazepine was prescribed for anxiety. Then Marian was asked to list all the stressors in her life and identify those she could and those she could not "fix." When the physician reviewed the list with her, the unavoidable stressors were reduced from a perceived 80% to about 30%. Marian was assisted in setting boundaries to establish her personal space and deflect stress from her environment. For example, one stressor was that her activity tripled when her grandchildren visited, resulting in unrelenting pain. By determining limits with those visits, Marian could prevent exceeding her capacity.

Stress management/relaxation techniques also were employed. As part of cognitive restructuring, Marian was taught an exercise to DEFOCUS–FOCUS–REFOCUS. She used her grandchildren in the exercise as follows:

DEFOCUS (how I feel—"back hurts")

FOCUS (concentrate on grandchildren)

REFOCUS (how I feel now—"good")

Methadone was ordered twice/day (9:00 A.M. and 9:00 P.M.). Methadone has particular advantage when opioids will be needed for many years, because significant pain relief can be achieved from small incremental dose increases. Marian will probably become habituated to methadone; however, she has a viable program for lifetime pain relief without the excessive dosages associated with other opioids (small increases every 6 months to 1 year).

Another reason for the choice of methadone was to achieve long-acting pain relief and break the cycle of dependence on medication. This, too, is imperative to cognitive restructuring, that is, changing the view of pain. Ineffective pain protocols result in the patient having pain, taking medication for the relief, and associating pain relief with the medication. Such cycles result in a dependence on medication and a belief that the pain can only be controlled externally. It is essential to change this thinking to a control mode. By obtaining reasonable pain relief through the twice-a-day dosing, Marian was able to associate pain relief and prevention during the day with her own interventions. When she experienced breakthrough pain about 2:00 P.M. daily, the evening dose was increased. Based on the long half-live of methadone, the strategy was to create a peak period in the afternoon (the prior-evening dose half-life combined with the morning-dose effects provided adequate coverage for the vulnerable afternoon period). Avoiding the introduction of another medication at time of breakthrough maintained the integrity of the self-control model. Although medications were employed, the real foundation of pain management was nonpharmacologic—i.e., placing Marian in control of her pain and her life. How much the patient does for him or herself determines success of pain relief, not how much medication is ordered.

In summary, chronic pain is a multidimensional phenomenon that can have a major impact on both the patient and his or her family. Effective therapy for this complex clinical challenge includes the family and addresses chronic pain management in a comprehensive manner. Clinicians must be sensitive to the burden of chronic pain and develop trusting relationships with the patient. The basis of therapy is nonpharmacologic, centered in the patient as the authority and controller of pain. Treatment is multimodal, and medications are used as supplemental rather than primary mechanisms. The goals of chronic pain relief should be to minimize discomfort and maximize function.

Clinical Accountabilities

1. Develop trust. Listen to the patient and be sensitive to his or her pain. Acceptance of the pain is acceptance of the patient.

2. Recognize that chronic pain itself is a complex disease state.
   - Chronicity reduces/eliminates physiologic evidence of pain.
   - Persistent pain leads to decreased functionality.
   - Prolonged pain often causes depression and despair.

3. Understand the multidimensionality of chronic pain. Appreciate that pain and the rest of the patient's life are inseparable.
   - Recognize and treat depression or anxiety caused by persistent pain and loss of self-esteem.
   - Identify lifestyle impact of physical limitations—social isolation, role changes in family.
   - Consider financial burden of lost work, increased medical expenses, search for "magic" medication or therapy.

4. Include the family, significant others throughout the process: assessment, planning, intervention, and evaluation phases.

5. Develop understanding of what is causing the pain, but be aware that often chronic pain persists after the pathology is eliminated.

6. Consider preexisting medical problems, medication regimens.

7. Set goals that improve quality of life.
   - Minimize pain, anxiety/depression.
   - Maximize functional level.

Continued on following page

Clinical Accountabilities *(Continued)*

8. Assist the patient in developing realistic expectations.
   - Elimination of pain may not be possible, but relief may be more feasible.
   - Activities may not be fully resumed. Question how adaptation can be accomplished while preserving greatest functionality.
   - Assist rethinking of self and adapting to a new role/identity if appropriate.

9. Put the patient in control, using cognitive restructuring. Ownership is key to pacing activities, setting boundaries, and ultimately obtaining pain relief.

10. Employ a multimodal approach with nonpharmacologic framework for pain management reinforced by pharmacologic use as appropriate.

11. Avoid pain/fear of pain cycle.
   - Medicate on scheduled basis, preferably using long-acting medications to break the cycle of dependence on medications for pain relief.
   - Dispel fear of addiction. Use opioids, adjunctive medications to relieve pain first, then establish a long-term plan.
   - Educate the patient on self-directed pain relief interventions.

12. Use a multidisciplinary approach with consistency from the whole health care team.
   - Ensure effective, consistent communications.
   - Establish optimal functioning through physical and occupational therapy.
   - Include social services for financial and social issues.
   - Refer to pain management teams or pain clinics as indicated.

BIBLIOGRAPHY

Baquie, M.L. (1989). What matters most in chronic pain management. *R.N.,* 46–50.

Bonica, J.J. (1990). *The management of pain* (2nd ed.). Philadelphia: Lea & Febiger.

Citera, J.A. (1992). The use of local anesthetics in the treatment of chronic pain. *Orthopedic Nursing, 11,* 27–33.

Copp, L.A., (1985). *Recent advances in nursing: Perspectives on pain.* Edinburgh: Churchill, Livingston.

Hitchcock, L., Ferrell, B., & McCaffery, M. (1994). The experience of chronic nonmalignant pain. *Journal of Pain and Symptom Management, 9*(5), 312–316.

Krause, S., Tiat, R., & Margolis, R. (1989). Pain distribution, intensity, and duration in patients with chronic pain. *Journal of Pain and Symptom Management, 9*(2), 67–71.

Malseed, R.T., & Wilson, B.A. (1993). Non-steroidal anti-inflammatory drugs in chronic pain. *MedSurg Nursing, 2*(2), 144–146.

Managing chronic pain with laser therapy. (1990–1991). *Canadian Critical Care Nursing Journal,* 6–7.

McCaffery, M. (1979). *Nursing management of the patient with pain.* Philadelphia: Lippincott.

McCaffery, M., & Beebe, A. (1989). *Pain: Clinical Manual for nursing practice.* St. Louis, MO: Mosby.

McCormack, G., Levine, M., Brown, G., Rangno, R., & Ruedy, J. (1996). *Drug therapy decision making guide.* Philadelphia: Saunders.

Owens, M.D., & Ehrenreich, D. (1991). Application of non-pharmacologic methods of managing chronic pain. *Holistic Nursing Practice, 6*(1), 32–40.

Portenoy, R. (1990). Chronic opioid therapy in non-malignant pain. *Journal of Pain and Symptom Management, 5*(1), 546–562.

Rose, K.E. (1994). Patient isolation in chronic benign pain. *Nursing standards, 8,* 51.

Schorr, J.A. (1993). Music and pattern change in chronic pain. *Advances in Nursing Science,* 17–36.

Snelling, J. (1994). The effect of chronic pain on the family unit. *Journal of Advanced Nursing, 19,* 543–551.

Strauss, A.L., & Glaser, B.G. (1975). *Chronic illness and the quality of life.* St. Louis, MO: Mosby.

Watt-Watson, J., & Donovan, M. (1992). *Pain management nursing perspective.* St. Louis, MO: Mosby Year Book.

10
Cancer and HIV/AIDS Pain

CANCER PAIN

Pain, one of the most feared consequences of the cancer experience, has been frequently undertreated in both adults and children. The National Cancer Institute *Workshop on Cancer Pain* (1990) articulated in its consensus statement that inadequate management was indeed a reality. Both national and international agencies, including the World Health Organization (WHO) and the Agency for Health Care Policy and Research, Department of Health and Human Services, have addressed the issue not only with policy statements but with well-researched clinical guidelines. Focused attention on the problem has resulted in abundant resources for the clinician who lacks the requisite knowledge and skill to manage this patient population. The bottom line is that most cancer pain can be well managed if clinicians use an aggressive approach that incorporates nonopioid and opioid analgesics and other appropriate nonpharmacologic interventions. In addition to the availability of sound clinical guidelines, there also is increasing societal permission to liberally, but appropriately, use opioid analgesics to manage the pain. Charles Cleeland and his colleagues in Wisconsin (1994) assessed the adequacy of cancer analgesic therapy in a large group of patients. They discovered that treatment was "adequate" in 85% of those surveyed. Although it is clear that focused attention on the problem in combination with excellent clinical guidelines has contributed to improved pain management for cancer patients, it is equally clear that much work remains to be done.

Cancer pain results from tumor progression and related pathology and/or treatment interventions

TABLE 10–1 *Classification of Cancer Pain*

CLASSIFICATION	IMPLICATIONS
Acute cancer related A. Associated with tumor burden B. Associated with cancer therapy	A. When pain is the precursor to the diagnosis of cancer, any future episodes, regardless of origin, provoke fear of disease recurrence B. Patients understand the pain's etiology and know it to be time-limited. Under these circumstances, individuals can frequently tolerate considerable discomfort
Chronic cancer related A. Associated with tumor progression B. Associated with cancer therapy	A. As increasing tumor burden escalates pain, doses increase and treatment may change. Anger, anxiety, depression, and a sense of helplessness can result. The pain becomes a constant reminder of the cancer's presence and immediacy of death B. As this type of pain may become chronic, it is imperative that the patient/family understand it is unrelated to the tumor

History of nonmalignant chronic pain	The diagnosis of cancer and its related pain can be yet another drain on available resources. Patients may already have compromised psychologic and functional states
History of substance abuse	Patients may require larger doses than those who are opioid-naive. There is an ethical obligation to treat the pain regardless of the patient's history
Terminal stage	Comfort is the primary goal. Pain can interrupt the patient/family's ability to communicate, to finish business, and to come to terms with impending death. Family and caregivers can be left with guilt and anger when those for whom they care die in unrelieved pain

(chemotherapy, biotherapy, radiation, surgery). On the average nearly 75% of patients with advanced cancer have pain. Forty percent to fifty percent describe it as moderate to severe, and 25% to 30% describe it as very severe (Bonica, 1990). Cancer pain can be excruciatingly comprehensive in its effects on the individual's quality of life and will impact physical, psychological, social, and spiritual domains (Ferrell et al., 1991). The physiologic demands and psychologic implications of the cancer pain experience make it difficult to categorize, but the simple classification offered in Table 10–1 can provide some insight into patient response to the experience.

Assessment

The assessment of cancer pain is based on the same principles as for assessing pain of any etiology. A thorough history and physical examination in conjunction with appropriate diagnostic tests may be used. Ultrasounds, MRIs, X-rays, CT scans, and bone scans can document primary and/or metastatic disease, pathologic fractures, and spinal cord compression. This diagnostic evaluation should include the signs and symptoms associated with the common cancer pain syndromes (bone and epidural metastases, spinal cord compression, plexopathies, and peripheral neuropathies). The patient interview should solicit the intensity and character of the pain, including onset, location, description, aggravating and relieving factors, and efficacy of previous treatment.

Assessment of cancer pain that is chronic in nature occurs on a continuum, and changes in the pattern or type of pain demand further evaluation. Cancer pain, with its many implications, further requires a thorough psychosocial assessment to determine its effect on the physical and social functioning of the patient and family. See Chapter 3 for more details.

Treatment

Multiple effective treatment options are available to manage cancer pain. There is not a single approach;

treatment modalities and psychosocial interventions are tailored to the individual's needs. The goal is to provide maximum pain relief with the least invasive modality possible. A combination of nonpharmacologic, psychologic, pharmacologic, surgical, neurosurgical, radiologic, and anesthetic interventions may be indicated.

Nonpharmacologic management can include physical modalities such as cutaneous stimulation (vibration, massage, use of heat and cold), exercise, immobilization, transcutaneous electrical nerve stimulation (TENS), and acupuncture. Although they offer some relief, these modalities should not be used as substitutes for pharmacologic intervention.

Psychologic interventions include, but are not limited to, relaxation and guided imagery, distraction and reframing, patient education, psychotherapy and structured support, hypnosis, peer support groups, and pastoral counseling. The complex nature and meaning of the pain experience require a multidimensional, multidisciplinary approach.

The primary cancer treatment modalities of surgery, chemotherapy, biologic response modifiers, or radiation therapy may be used, but do not routinely provide total relief. Surgical and neurosurgical procedures include tumor debulking, relieving spinal cord compression, orthopedic procedures for stabilizing bony structures, and neuroablative procedures. Chemotherapy may be used in an effort to shrink the tumor.

Radiation therapy when used palliatively for pain relief is less intense and of shorter duration than that used for primary treatment of the tumor. It may be localized or cover a wide field, is intended to shrink tumor in soft tissues or bone, and may significantly decrease metastatic pain as well as pain from local extension of primary disease. Tumor metastatic to the bone is a primary target for palliative radiation therapy. Pain relief may result from the prevention of pathologic fractures or the promotion of health in an already established fracture. Radiation therapy also may alleviate painful nerve compression or infiltration by tumor. *Brachytherapy,* or the placement of a radioactive source within the tissue to deliver localized radiation, may be used to treat recurrent disease previously treated by external beam therapy and can assist in relieving localized pain.

Radiopharmaceuticals such as Iodine-131 and strontium-89 are but two examples of therapeutic agents used to treat pain resulting from multiple bone metastases. They are administered intravenously and will act directly upon sites of metastatic deposit in the bone. Aredia®, a bone resorption inhibitor, has demonstrated a significant reduction in bone pain with a 90 mg dose administered monthly via an intravenous line.

Anesthetic interventions include temporary and permanent neural blockades and catheter placement for drug delivery in the epidural or intrathecal space. Neurosurgical procedures may also be indicated for the rare few for whom less invasive methods have been unsuccessful. See further discussion of spinal analgesia in Chapter 5.

The majority of cancer pain is relieved pharmacologically. The World Health Organization Relief Program has formulated an analgesic ladder using nonopioid, opioid, and adjuvant analgesics alone or in combination for the treatment of cancer pain. This escalating pharmacotherapeutic approach begins with the nonopioid analgesics for mild to moderate pain, adds an opioid such as codeine or oxycodone with or without an adjuvant analgesic as the pain increases, and ultimately recommends an opioid such as morphine, hydromorphone (Dilaudid®), levorphanol (Levo-Dromoran®), or methadone (Dolophine®) in combination with nonopioid analgesics and adjuvant medications to treat severe pain (Figure 10-1).

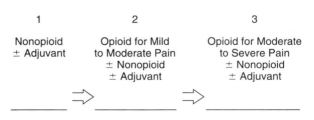

1	2	3
Nonopioid ± Adjuvant	Opioid for Mild to Moderate Pain ± Nonopioid ± Adjuvant	Opioid for Moderate to Severe Pain ± Nonopioid ± Adjuvant

FIGURE 10–1 *WHO's Three-Step Analgesic Ladder*

Principles of Analgesic Therapy

Drug Selection

1. Begin with the mildest agents that control the pain. Use a multidrug approach. The use of nonopioids and adjuvant analgesics may increase analgesic efficacy and allow a decreased opioid dosage.

2. When nonopioid and mild opioid analgesics administered simultaneously at the maximally tolerated or recommended dosage are ineffective, proceed to a more potent opioid.

3. It is unnecessary to use analgesic combinations with fixed-ratio formulas (e.g., Percocet®, Tylenol #3®). The nonopioid and opioid components can be titrated individually to meet the patient's needs.

4. Consider the drug's side effect profile. For instance, if the patient has a history of peptic ulcer disease, thrombocytopenia, or is currently receiving ulcerogenic medications, select a nonopioid that does not markedly effect platelet aggregation or the gastrointestinal mucosa.

5. Select an alternative nonopioid if one particular choice is ineffective. As the nonsteroidal anti-inflammatory drugs (NSAIDs) differ in chemical structure, patients may respond very well to an alternative choice.

6. Do not combine the nonopioids. There is an increased risk of gastric and renal toxicity. An exception is acetaminophen, which may be given safely with NSAIDs.

7. Use as first-line agents the pure agonist opioids (oxycodone, codeine, morphine, hydromorphone, methadone, levorphanol, and fentanyl). Although it is an opioid agonist, meperidine is not recommended for chronic use because of the accumulation of its active metabolite, normeperidine, which can cause central nervous system (CNS) excitatory effects (Kaiko et al., 1983).

8. Unmanageable toxicities secondary to opioid

analgesics may be ameliorated in some patients by selecting another opioid at an equianalgesic dosage.

9. Avoid the agonist-antagonist opioids (pentazocine, nalbuphine, butorphanol, and buprenorphine). They are not suitable for pain requiring significant analgesic doses.

10. Use opioid analgesics that have a short half-life for breakthrough pain. If possible, use the same drug as the scheduled analgesic.

11. Utilize the atypical analgesics (e.g. antidepressants, anticonvulsants) for patients with neuropathic pain not controlled by opioid analgesics alone.

12. Do not use placebos to assess the nature of the pain. An analgesic effect from placebo does not furnish the clinician any practical information about the severity of the pain (American Pain Society, 1992).

Dosage Titration/Scheduling

1. Use scheduled dosing as the standard. This maintains even serum levels of the drug and can provide consistent relief. Scheduled dosing does not preclude the need for treating breakthrough pain **(rescue dosing).**

2. Consider rescue dosing alone when the analgesic dosage is uncertain, during initial titration of opioids with a long half-life (e.g., methadone) or during therapy that may markedly decrease the analgesic dosage (e.g., radiation therapy for bone metastases).

3. Provide rescue dosing on an as-needed basis, and increase or decrease the dose depending on the analgesic effects.

4. Adjust the scheduled dose if frequent rescue dosing is required. The cumulative rescue dose used in a 24-hour period should be divided by the number of times the scheduled medication is administered in that time period and added to the scheduled dose.

5. Base the administration schedule on the analgesic's duration of effect. Immediate release and timed-release preparations can be scheduled accordingly.

6. Once significant pain relief is achieved, maintain that dosage for four to five half-lives of the drug to reach steady serum plasma levels and evaluate the complete analgesic effect (Portenoy, 1992).

7. Use equianalgesic dosage principles. See Tables 4-4 and 4-5 in Chapter 4. When changing to a drug with a similar duration of effect, begin with a dose that is one-half to two-thirds the equianalgesic dose of the current medication as cross tolerance is not complete (American Pain Society, 1992).

8. When converting to controlled-release morphine preparations, use approximately two-thirds of the prior daily dose. Continue to provide rescue dosing immediate-release analgesics equivalent to about one-sixth of the 24-hour total to be given every 2 hours as needed (American Pain Society, 1992).

9. Be aware of tolerance (increased dosing necessary to control the same amount of pain). Strategies to forestall tolerance include using the oral route of administration, maximizing analgesia by using a combination of nonopioid and opioid agents, and selecting another opioid.

10. Taper the opioid slowly for patients requiring a lesser dosage. Chronic exposure to opioids does produce physical dependence, and sudden cessation will produce signs and symptoms of withdrawal (agitation, tremors, insomnia, fear, autonomic nervous system hyperexcitability, and increased pain).

KEY POINT

Cancer pain is chronic in nature and requires, with rare exception, both scheduled and rescue dosing.

Route/Method of Administration

1. Use an appropriate route of administration based on physiologic needs, patient comfort and preference, and caregiver capacity. Many patients over the disease continuum will require a change in the route of administration.

2. Use the route that minimizes drug concentration at the site producing the side effect (e.g., a nonoral route is preferable for patients with partial bowel obstruction to eliminate significant opioid levels in the stomach and intestine).

3. Use the route that can effectively provide relief promptly. Severe, escalating pain requires immediate attention. Intravenous (IV) administration has the most rapid onset of action. IV opioids may be given by intermittent injections, continuous infusion, or a combination of the two. Patient-controlled analgesia (PCA) pumps have been used effectively to titrate the analgesic dosage to desired effect.

4. Intramuscular and subcutaneous injections are painful and provide inconsistent absorption at best. Low-volume subcutaneous infusions may be very effective when IV access is unavailable or impractical.

5. Epidural and intrathecal opioids can provide excellent relief for specified patient populations. See Chapter 5 for further information.

6. The oral route is the preferred one. If the dose and schedule are correct, oral opioids can be as effective as parenteral opioids.

7. Be aware of the equianalgesic differences of the varied routes. The **first-pass effect** of hepatic metabolism requires higher oral dosing of opioid agents than when those same agents are administered parenterally.

Side Effect Management

1. There is tremendous variation in individual susceptibility to opioid-mediated side effects.

Careful monitoring should accompany initiation of therapy. Respiratory depression can occur in opioid-naive individuals and those with pulmonary disease but is uncommon with careful titration. Hypersensitivity reactions are rare. If they occur, use an opioid from another subclass.

2. Sedation is not uncommon with initial opioid therapy. Tolerance soon develops in most patients.

3. Constipation occurs routinely with opioid use, and patients do not develop tolerance to this side effect. A prophylactic bowel regimen is recommended.

4. The use of opioid antagonists such as naloxone (Narcan®) to reverse harmful opioid effects also can reverse analgesia and precipitate acute withdrawal. Opioid antagonists are not recommended to reverse non–life-threatening effects, such as confusion or sedation. When used to reverse life-threatening respiratory depression or hypotension, they should be diluted and titrated to effect. See Chapter 4 for further details.

CASE STUDY

Margaret is a 54-year-old female with recurrent metastatic breast cancer. She was treated with chemotherapy 3 years before and appeared to be in remission until approximately 6 weeks ago. She presented with diffuse bony metastases in the spine and pelvic region. She is afraid to move around because her pain increases to excruciating levels. She reports her pain to be a 9 on a scale of 0 to 10. While hospitalized for a metastatic workup, she was given 4 mg morphine IV every 15 minutes as needed for pain. In the first 8 hours of therapy, she requires 10 doses of morphine. With her current needs documented at 5 mg morphine/hour, she is placed on a continuous morphine infusion at 5 mg/hour. The physician also orders an NSAID on a scheduled basis and 5 mg morphine IV every hour as needed for breakthrough pain. During the following 16 hours Margaret requires only three rescue doses of 5 mg each. Her total 24-hour parenteral morphine requirements equal 135 mg. The physician makes the parenteral/oral conversion calculation at 1 mg:3 mg. She is prescribed a controlled-release morphine preparation at 130 mg every 8 hours. The physician also orders rescue dosing for breakthrough pain of morphine 15 mg sublingually every 1 hour as needed. He continues 600 mg Motrin® four times a day.

Twenty-four hours into her oral analgesic therapy, Margaret has required only 2 rescue doses. Both instances centered on getting out of bed to the chair. The nurse suggests that Margaret use a sublingual morphine tablet at least 20 to 30 minutes before attempting activity to determine whether the ordered dosage is effective for incident pain. Several hours later she wished to sit in her bedside chair, and the sublingual morphine was administered. After waiting 25 minutes, Margaret got out of bed with minimal discomfort. She reported to the nurse that her pain seemed to be under control. She went on to say that she wasn't sleeping very well. The pain no longer kept her awake, but she couldn't seem to shut her mind off. Her nurse contacted the physician and requested a mild sleeping intervention and a social services consult. Benadryl® 25 mg at bedtime was ordered. The LCSW spent an hour with Margaret. She verbalized her concern for the future, what would happen to her house, how she would manage as she became progressively more ill, who would take care of her. The social worker provided assistance with her financial problems and discussed her concerns with the physician. Margaret was referred to a home health agency for her immediate discharge nursing needs, and the social worker initiated a discussion of hospice care. Margaret took great comfort in this discussion and began to plan in an organized way. She continued to be managed on the oral morphine preparations, Motrin® and Benadryl® very effectively until discharge.

HIV/AIDS PAIN

As has been historically true for cancer pain, pain in the AIDS population is widespread, undermanaged, and has a significant impact on the patient's quality of life. Disease progression equals increased pain, and AIDS patients typically present with two or three different kinds of pain at any one time. Patient subsets include the female population whose pain is common and even more dramatically undertreated and the pediatric population whose pain is infrequently identified and customarily undertreated. The most common pediatric pain syndromes include headache due to CNS, meningeal, and sinus infections; pain due to skin infections; abdominal pain and oral pain; and extremity pain associated with extreme spasticity in children with late stages of AIDS dementia complex. Although the AIDS pain experience is remarkably similar to the cancer pain experience, it is distinguished by the fact that the pain is much more dramatically undertreated.

Pain syndromes in the AIDS population occur secondary to the virus and its sequelae or as a direct result of therapeutic interventions. Common pain manifestations include: (1) neuropathic pain syndromes (e.g., HIV-induced polyneuropathy, myelopathy secondary to viral infections of the spinal cord, and peripheral neuropathy due to the neurotoxic effects of alcohol abuse); (2) chest pain (retrosternal burning related to pneumocystis carinii pneumonia); (3) esophageal and oral cavity pain (secondary to candidiasis and herpes simplex); (4) pain secondary to extensive Kaposi's sarcoma involving soft-tissue invasion, edema, and secondary infection; (5) pain from infectious processes; (6) abdominal pain related to infection, diarrhea, organomegaly, and obstruction; (7) rheumatologic syndromes; (8) headaches (secondary to HIV-related involvement of the CNS, primary CNS lymphoma, toxoplasmosis or as a result of azidothymidine therapy); and (9) treatment-related neuropathies secondary to exposure to DDI, DDC, D4T, rifampin, and pentamadine.

Pain in the AIDS and cancer patient populations is equally multidimensional and complex, and treatment principles are similar. The demands of physical, emotional, and socioenvironmental factors require a multidisciplinary, multimodal pain management approach. In the AIDS population there seems to be a strong correlation between perceived intensity of pain and disease progression. Those who view their pain as evidence of increasing pathology report it to be more severe than patients who see no connection between their pain experience and disease progression.

Recommended pain management approaches include treating any correctable cause of pain with surgery, antiviral, antifungal, or antibiotic agents and treating pain as a symptom when the etiology cannot be effectively eradicated. A basic premise of AIDS pain management comes from the cancer pain management model. The World Health Organization analgesic ladder that has become the standard for cancer pain management also serves this patient population well. Analgesic therapies are chosen based on the intensity and type of pain. This stairstep approach beginning with nonopioid analgesics and/or atypical analgesics and escalating to opioid preparations in combination with nonopioids and/or atypical analgesics as the pain increases in intensity should become the standard for AIDS pain management as well.

As outlined in Chapter 4, nonopioid, opioid, and atypical analgesic preparations are used for pain management. They are suitable choices for both the chronic and acute pain that may occur over the AIDS disease continuum. When pain levels are mild, a nonopioid preparation (e.g., acetaminophen or an NSAID) may be adequate. As the pain intensity increases and opioid preparations are required, there may be extraordinary dosage requirements in some patients, such as those with a history of substance abuse. If the patient is an active opioid user or on a methadone maintenance program, sufficient drug must be given to overcome tolerance to the usual opioid level. Short-acting opioids are appropriate for unpredictable or breakthrough pain, and longer-acting opioids are used for chronic pain. Patients with advanced HIV disease receiving medications that act centrally, including opioid therapy, should be carefully monitored because they are especially susceptible to confusion or delirium. Other side effects common to opioid preparations require the same attention and treatment as for any other patient population.

The neuropathic syndromes common in the AIDS population are treated with atypical analgesics (e.g., antidepressants and anticonvulsants) in combination with opioid preparations. Antidepressants used for analgesic purposes (e.g., amitriptyline, desipramine, nortriptyline) require dosage fine-tuning. Recent evidence suggests that there may be less difference between analgesic and antidepressant dosages than previously surmised, and thus the antidepressant dosage should be titrated upward to effect. Pain may begin to improve 4 to 6 days into therapy. Anticonvulsants commonly chosen for neuropathic syndromes characterized by shooting, lancinating pain include carbamazepine (Tegretol®), clonazepam (Klonopin®), and valproic acid (Depakene®). See Chapter 4 for further details.

In summary, the basic tenets of AIDS pain management are similar to the cancer pain management model. The clinician should use a multidisciplinary, multimodal approach; treat underlying causes of the pain when possible; and use nonopioid, opioid, and atypical analgesic interventions based on the character and intensity of the pain.

ROLE AND RESPONSIBILITY OF THE NURSE

Nurses play a vital role in the management of cancer and HIV pain. Frequent access to the patient provides a unique opportunity to evaluate pain status and response to pain-relieving measures. A thorough knowledge of pain management principles prepares the nurse to serve as an effective collaborator on the health care team. Ongoing assessment and a sound knowledge base position the nurse to function competently as the patient's advocate. One of the most important interventions centers on bias about or inadequate knowledge of the use of opioid analgesics. Other health care team members as well as the patient may fear the possibilities of overdosage and/or addiction. It is of paramount importance that at least one clinician articulate management principles and goals and be able to provide practical recommendations for meeting those goals.

The varied and complex physical and psychosocial stressors common to these patient populations require knowledgeable, compassionate caregivers. Pain is a reality throughout the disease continuum for the majority of patients and deserves the full attention of the health care team.

Clinical Accountabilities

1. Have a thorough understanding of basic pain management strategies.
   - Principles of drug selection and dosing.
   - Equianalgesia and parenteral/oral conversion methods.
   - Advantages/disadvantages of varied routes of administration.
   - Nonopioid, opioid, and atypical analgesic side effect management.

2. Assess pain systematically.
   - Evaluate effectiveness after each dose until pain is well controlled.
   - Base assessment on the patient's report.
   - Use the same quantitative assessment method consistently.
   - Reassess thoroughly when the patient's pain has changed or is escalating rapidly.

3. Function as the patient's advocate.
   - Contact the physician when the patient is not receiving adequate relief from ordered interventions.
   - Provide an articulate and concise assessment, including the intensity, location, and nature of the sensation and the response to ordered analgesics (drug, dosage, and route with amount and duration of relief).
   - Offer suggestions for dosage or medication alternatives.
   - Continue collaboration with the physician until the patient is comfortable at an identified dosage and interval.
   - Question the use of placebos.

Clinical Accountabilities *(Continued)*

4. Utilize knowledge of drug selection, dosage titration, and scheduling principles.
   - Choose the appropriate analgesic when more than one is ordered.
   - Be aware of nonopioid side effects when treating a patient with thrombocytopenia or a history of peptic ulcer disease.
   - Consider the atypical analgesics for patients with neuropathic pain.
   - Monitor ordered analgesics for incompatibility.

5. Clarify orders and collaborate with the physician when:
   - An agonist-antagonist opioid or meperidine is ordered for long-term use
   - Scheduled and/or rescue analgesic orders are not provided
   - The scheduled analgesic is ordered at an interval greater than the drug's duration of effect
   - Frequent rescue dosing is necessary in addition to the scheduled analgesic
   - Controlled-release opioid preparations are ordered as needed or at a less than 8-hour interval.
   - Conversion to an alternative route or medication is not based on equianalgesic knowledge.
   - The route of chronic opioid administration is intramuscular.
   - The ordered route becomes inadequate or inappropriate.
   - An opioid antagonist is ordered to counteract sedation that is not life-threatening.

6. Anticipate and treat side effects.
   - Prophylactically treat anticipated constipation secondary to opioid analgesics.
   - Administer antiemetics prophylactically during initial opioid therapy.
   - As opioid dosing increases be alert for signs of myoclonus or any other CNS toxicity.

Continued on following page

Clinical Accountabilities *(Continued)*

7. Educate the patient/family/significant other/care-giver.
   - Right to and benefit of adequate analgesia.
   - Patient's role in and importance of accurate assessment.
   - Analgesic side effects and their management.
   - Address misconceptions/fears of physical depen-dence, tolerance, and psychological dependence.
   - Develop contractual agreements for opioid use in patients with a history of substance abuse.

8. Document assessment and interventions.
   - Provide an accurate and clear record of the nature, location, and intensity of the pain.
   - Consistently report the results of ordered inter-ventions.

BIBLIOGRAPHY

American Pain Society. (1992). *Principles of analgesic use in the treatment of acute pain and cancer pain* (3rd ed.). Skokie, IL: American Pain Society.

Bonica, J.J. (1990). Cancer pain. In J.J. Bonica (Ed.), *The management of pain* (2nd ed., pp. 400–460). Philadelphia: Lea & Febiger.

Breitbart, W. (1996). Pain management and psychosocial issues in HIV and AIDS. *The American Journal of Hospice & Palliative Care,* January/February, 20–29.

Cleeland, C.S., Gonin, R., Hatfield, A.K., Edmonson, J.H., Blum, R.H., Steward, J.A., & Pandya, K.J. (1994). Pain and its treatment in outpatients with metastatic cancer. *New England Journal of Medicine 3,* 592–596.

De Stoutz, N.D., Bruera, E., & Suarez-Almazor, M. (1995). Opioid rotation for toxicity reduction in terminal cancer patients. *Journal of Pain and Symptom Management, 10*(5), 378–384.

Ferrell, B.R., Rhiner, M., Cohen, M.Z., & Grant, M. (1991). Pain as a metaphor for illness. Part II: Family caregivers' management of pain. *Oncology Nursing Forum, 18*(8), 1303–1309.

Jacox, A., Carr, D.B., and Payne, R., et al. (1994). *Management of cancer pain. Clinical practice guideline.* ACHPR Publication No. 94-0592. Rockville, MD: Agency for Health Care Policy and Research, U.S. Department of Health and Human Services.

Kaiko, R.F., Foley, K.M., Grabinski, P.Y., Heidrick, G., Rogers, A.G., Inturrisi, C.E., & Reidenberg, M.M. (1983). Central nervous system excitatory effects of meperidine in cancer patients. *Annals of Neurology, 13*(2), 180–185.

Miser, A.W., Dothage, J.A., Wesley, R.A., & Miser, J.S. The prevalence of pain in a pediatric and young adult cancer population. *Clinical Journal of Pain, 29*(1), 73–83.

National Cancer Institute. (1990). *NCI Workshop on Cancer Pain.* Bethesda, MD: National Cancer Institute.

Paice, J.A. (1996). Pain. In Groenwald, S.L., Frogge, M.H., Goodman, M., & Yarbro, C.H. (Eds.), *Cancer symptom management.* Needham: Jones & Bartlett.

Patt, R.B. (1993). *Cancer pain.* Philadelphia: Lippincott.

Penfold, J., & Clark, A.J.M. (1992). Pain syndromes in HIV infection. *Canadian Journal of Anaesthesia, 39*(7), 724–730.

Portenoy, R.K. (1992). Pain management in the older cancer patient. *Oncology, 6* (Supp. 2), 86–98.

Sande, M.A., & Volberding, P.A. (1995). *The medical management of AIDS.* (4th ed.). Philadelphia: Saunders.

Spross, J.A., McGuire, D.B., & Schmitt, R.M. (1990). Oncology nursing society position paper on cancer pain. *Oncology Nursing Forum 17*(4–6). 595–614, 751–760, 943–955.

World Health Organization. (1990). *Cancer pain relief and palliative care. Report of a WHO expert committee.* World Health Organization Technical Report Series, 804. Geneva, Switzerland: World Health Organization.

11
Pain in Infants and Children

The assessment, treatment, and evaluation of pain in children is a component of nursing practice that deserves special attention. Unfortunately, children suffer needlessly because the concepts of pediatric pain management often are misunderstood, ignored, or unnoticed. Children are unique individuals, whose world does not accommodate models of adult-oriented care. There is a need for age-specific, developmentally focused care. Neonatal pain management, especially in the premature infant, is in its evolutionary phase and lacks sufficient research to recommend any guidelines for management. Tools for assessment are not yet developed, tested, or accepted. For this reason neonatal pain management will not be discussed in this chapter. It is important to recognize, however, that infants experience pain and pain assessment in that population deserves attention.

Although age-appropriate pain assessment tools and developmentally appropriate approaches should be followed, the management of chronic pain in children is very similar to that of adults (see Chapter 9).

OUTDATED BELIEFS

A number of outdated beliefs continue to have currency. These include:

- Neonates and infants do not feel pain at all.
- Children do not feel pain with the same intensity as adults.
- Children become accustomed to pain and tolerate discomfort well.

- Children have no memory of pain.
- Children tell you if they are in pain.
- Children always tell the truth about pain.
- Children are not in pain if they can be distracted or they are sleeping.
- Parents exaggerate their child's pain.
- PRN medication orders mean that medication should be given as infrequently as possible.
- Postoperative pain medications should not be administered until obvious signs of pain are exhibited.
- The best route for giving analgesics is intramuscular.
- Nurses prefer intravenous administration over intramuscular administration because it is more convenient for them.
- Respiratory depression and addiction are dangerous side effects in pediatric pain management.

Although research exists to disprove all of these fallacies, a substantial number of health care professionals continue to base their pain management practices on such outdated beliefs. It is imperative that nurses gain knowledge of proper pain assessment to advocate for appropriate management of pediatric pain.

PRINCIPLES OF PAIN ASSESSMENT

Physiologic responses to pain among children are similar to adult responses and include flushing of the skin; increases in heart rate, blood pressure, and respiratory rate; decreases in oxygen saturation levels; fluctuations in intracranial pressure; restlessness; sweating; and dilation of the pupils. It is important to note, however, that in children, these same physiologic changes may be evoked in response to fear, anxiety, parental separation and anger, and further evaluation should always take place.

Assessment of pain in children is complex and is compounded by constant physical and developmental flux. Health care providers must assess a child's pain not by adult criteria, but by using factors that influence the pain experience in children. The child's developmental level is an extremely important variable (Table 11–1).

Assessing a Child's Previous Pain Experience

Obtaining a child's pain history is an excellent method for assessing, planning, and evaluating appropriate pain management interventions. Children's verbal statements and descriptions of pain are the *most important* factors in assessing pain (Wong, 1995). Involving parents in this process will provide valuable insight into the child's coping strategies and developmental level (Table 11–2).

Pediatric Pain Assessment Tools

Numerous pain assessment scales have been developed to assess pain in children. Pain assessment tools can be categorized as those that elicit the child's self-report of pain and those that provide a format for nurses' observations of the child's behavior. Although many pain assessment tools exist, pediatric health care settings should rely only on those that have been researched for validity and reliability (Table 11–3).

PRINCIPLES OF NURSING MANAGEMENT

To provide effective nursing management of children in pain, health care providers must recognize the child's right to pain control. Nurses have an ethical obligation to relieve a child's suffering not only because of the consequences of unrelieved pain, but also because appropriate pain management may have further benefits, such as autonomy, control over stressful situations, shortened hospital stays, and

TABLE 11-1 *Guidelines for Age-Appropriate Pain Assessment*

Age	Behavioral Response to Painful Stimuli
Infant	
<6 months	Facial grimacing, cries vigorously, generalized body movements, chin quivering
6–12 months	Irritability, restlessness, thrashing, eyes tightly closed, local reflex withdrawal, disturbed sleep patterns
Toddler (1–3 years)	Cries, screams, struggles against restraint, difficult to comfort, may regress behaviorally, may verbalize "hurt" or "owee," established sleep patterns disturbed
Preschooler (3–5 years)	Cries, screams, struggles against restraint, directed aggressive behavior, strikes out physically and verbally when hurt, low frustration level, decreased interest in environment and usual activities
School-age children	
6–9 years	Passive resistance, clenches fists, engages in plea bargaining, cries, screams, localizes pain verbally, holds rigidly still
10–12 years	May pretend comfort to act brave, readily verbalizes complaints, concerns and protests, describes pain intensity, helps evaluate pain management interventions
Adolescents (13+ years)	Facial grimacing, muscular rigidity, may grunt, groan, or cry, voice quality may change, becoming soft or whiny, sleep disturbances, irritable, demanding

Adapted from Ball, J., & Bindler, R. (1995). *Pediatric nursing: Caring for children.* Norwalk, CT: Appleton & Lange; and Foster, R., & Stevens, B. (1994). Nursing management of pain in children. In C. Betz, M. Hunsberger, & S. Wright (Eds.), *Family-centered nursing care of children* (pp. 882–914). Philadelphia: Saunders.

TABLE 11–2   *Pain Experience History*

Child Form	Parent Form
Tell me what pain is.	What word(s) does your child use in regard to pain?
Tell me about the hurt you have had before.	Describe the pain experiences your child has had before.
Do you tell others when you hurt? If yes, who?	Does your child tell you or others when he or she is hurting?
What do you do for yourself when you are hurting?	How do you know when your child is in pain?
What do you want others to do for you when you hurt?	How does your child usually react to pain?
What don't you want others to do for you when you hurt?	What do you do for your child when he or she is hurting?
What helps the most to take your hurt away?	What does your child do for himself or herself when he or she is hurting?
Is there anything special that you want me to know about you when you hurt? (If yes, have child describe.)	What works best to decrease or take away your child's pain?
	Is there anything special that you would like me to know about your child and pain? (If yes, describe.)

Hester, N., & Barcus, C. (1986). Assessment and management of pain in children. *Pediatrics: Nursing Update,* Princeton, N.J.: Continuing Education Center 1, 2–8.

reduced costs. Nursing management involves the following:

- Recognition of pain and formulation of a nursing diagnosis
- Pharmacologic intervention
- Nonpharmacologic intervention

TABLE 11-3 *Selected Pediatric Pain Assessment Scales*

SCALE	AGE GROUP	ADMINISTRATION	USE
Eland Color Tool	4–9 years	You need six crayons: black, purple, blue, red, green, and orange; no one color is most often selected by children as representing the most pain; limited reliability and validity data	Child picks a crayon color representing the most pain, then color of next most pain, etc., until four crayons are selected; then child colors the body outline to indicate the location of the areas of hurt by level of pain
Oucher Scale	3–7 years	Child selects face that best fits his or her level of pain; older child selects a number between 0 and 100	Useful in hospital settings; child must understand concepts of higher/lower and more/less; cultural versions available; tool has been successfully tested for reliability and validity in some age groups
Poker Chip Scale	4–18 years	Child selects the number of red poker chips (0–4) that corresponds to level of hurt	Useful in any setting; inexpensive, easy to transport and clean
Adolescent Pediatric Pain Tool	8 years–adolescence	Child draws on front and back body outlines to locate pain; uses word graphic rating to indicate intensity and circles words to describe quality	Helpful in diagnosing pain syndromes and changes in pain parameters over time

Reprinted with permission: Eland Color Tool and Oucher Scale: Ball, J. & Bindler, R. (1995). *Pediatric Nursing: Caring for Children*, (p. 186), Norwalk, CT: Appleton & Lange. Oucher Scale: Beyer, Judith E. Poker Chip Scale developed in 1975 by Nancy O. Hester, University of Colorado Health Sciences Center, Denver, CO; Savedra, M., Tesler, M., Holzemer, W., & Ward, J. (1989). *Adolescent pediatric pain tool (APPT): Preliminary user's manual.* San Francisco: University of California.

- Monitoring the effectiveness of pain control interventions
- Patient/family education

Recognition

The goals of pain assessment are to (1) identify pain whenever it exists; and (2) obtain the best possible understanding of the location, intensity, and quality of pain (Foster & Stevens, 1994). Using baseline assessment strategies such as pain assessment tools, parent interview, child observation, and physiologic monitoring will help achieve these goals.

Pharmacologic Intervention

Acute pain in children is managed with nonsteroidal anti-inflammatory drugs (NSAIDs), opioid analgesics, and local anesthetics. Tables 11–4 and 11–5 outline common drugs used for pediatric pain management.

Administering analgesics to children is different from administering pain medications to adults because it is more difficult to determine the relative dose of medication being given. Whereas adult doses of narcotics and other analgesics usually vary only moderately among patients, doses for children are based *individually* on body weight and vary with each kilogram of difference in weight (Foster & Stevens, 1994). Safe calculation of pediatric drug dosages requires an understanding of the recommended therapeutic dose (Table 11–6).

Intramuscular Route

Appropriate pain management should rarely include the use of intramuscular (IM) injections. IM injection is a poor choice for narcotic administration because (1) altered tissue perfusion leads to unpredictable drug absorption and patient response; (2) there are limited number of injection sites; and (3) injections cannot be performed in children with thrombocytopenia (Burokas, 1985).

TABLE 11-4 *Common Pediatric Pain Medications*

Drug	Dose	Comments
Acetaminophen (many brand names, e.g., Tempra®, Tylenol®)	PO: 10–15 mg/kg q 4–6 hr Maximum: 4 gm, or 5 doses/24 hr	Lacks the peripheral anti-inflammatory activity of NSAIDs Available as oral liquid
Ibuprofen (many brand names, e.g., Children's Advil®, Pediaprofen®)	PO: 4–10 mg/kg q 6–8 hr Maximum: 40–60 mg/kg/24 hr	Inhibits production of prostaglandins, which mediate inflammation and pain Should be used short-term (48–72 hr) in post-operative patients
Ketorolac (Toradol®)	IV: 0.5–1 mg/kg as a single dose	Does not produce respiratory depression or sedation; very costly Suitable for moderate pain
Codeine	0.5–1 mg/kg PO/IM q 4–6 hr Parenteral route not recommended	Not intended for IV use because of histamine release and cardiovascular effects
Meperidine (Demerol®)	PO/SQ/IM/IV (over 5–10 min.): 1–1.5 mg/kg q 3–4 hr Maximum single dose: 100 mg	Toxic metabolite-normeperidine can cause seizures and dysphoria (with prolonged administration)
Morphine (Duramorph®, MS Contin®, MSIR®, Roxanol®)	*Infants:* SQ/IM/IV (slow): 0.05–0.2 mg/kg q 4 hr *Children:* SQ/IM/IV: 0.1–0.2 mg/kg q 2–4 hr Maximum Dose: 15 mg PO: 0.2–0.5 mg/kg q 4–6 hr PO (sustained release): 0.3–0.6 mg/kg q 12 hr	Respiratory depression may be exaggerated in the first 3 to 6 months of life

Hydromorphone (Dilaudid®)	IV: 0.015 mg/kg/dose q 4-6 hr Continuous infusion: Titrate dose as needed	Roughly 8-10 times as potent as morphine
Fentanyl (Sublimaze®)	IM/IV: 0.5-4 µg/kg q 2-4 hr or as continuous IV infusion of 1-3 µg/kg/hr	Higher doses used during anesthesia and in intensive care settings Similar to morphine (50-100 times as potent)
Midazolam (Versed®)	*Pre-Op Sedation:* PO: 0.4-0.5 mg/kg IM: 0.05-0.1 mg/kg IV (over 2-3 min.): 0.035 mg/kg *Conscious Sedation:* IV: Initially 0.05-0.2 mg/kg loading dose then IV infusion of 1-2 mcg/kg/hr Titrated to desired effect	Higher doses used during anesthesia and in intensive care settings Used as a sedative, amnesiac, and anxiolytic For painful procedures, should be accompanied by an opioid. Monitor heart rate, respiratory rate, and oxygen saturation carefully
EMLA® (eutectic mixture of local anesthetics) Topical anesthetic	2-2.5 gm is the recommended dose for infants >1 mo and children	Mixture of Lidocaine + Prilocaine Must be placed on intended puncture site and covered with an occlusive dressing for 60 minutes before the procedure

Note: Mixtures known as "DPT cocktails" (Demerol, Phenergan, Thorazine) are unsuitable for pediatric pain management and sedation purposes. The safety and efficacy of DPT does not compare favorably with the combination of opioids and benzodiazedines and should be used only under exceptional circumstances.

Reference: Taketomo, C., Hodding, J., & Kraus, D. (1996). *Pediatric dosage handbook* (3rd ed.). Cleveland, OH: Lexi-Comp.

203

TABLE 11-5 *Reversal Agents*

Drug	Common Pediatric Pain Medications	Comments
Naloxone (Narcan®)	*Respiratory depression due to opioids:* SQ/IM/IV: Initial dose is 0.01 mg/kg IV; give a subsequent dose of 0.1 mg/kg if needed. SQ or IM routes may be used if IV route not available.	Reverses most effects of opioids: sedation, respiratory depression, itching, and analgesia Individual titration is necessary
Flumazenil (Romazicon®)	*Reversal conscious sedation/anesthesia:* IV (over 1–2 min.): 0.01 mg/kg followed by 0.005-0.01 mg/kg every min. as needed up to maximum cumulative dose of 1 mg Maximum single dose: 0.2 mg *Benzodiazepine overdose:* IV: 0.01 mg/kg followed by 0.01 mg/kg every minute to a maximum cumulative dose of 1 mg	Reverses many effects of benzodiazepines May precipitate seizures in benzodiazepine-dependent patients

TABLE 11–6   *Calculation of Medication Ordered Based on Recommended Therapeutic Dose*

---

1. Determine the maximal recommended therapeutic dose for the drug
2. Determine the child's weight in kilograms (usually available on the nursing admission history)
3. Calculate the maximal therapeutic dose
   Example:
   Drug: Codeine elixir
   Maximal recommended therapeutic dose: 1 mg/kg q3–4 hr (Acute Pain Management Guideline Panel, 1992)
   Child's weight: 30 kg
   Maximal dose for this child: 1 mg × 30 kg = 30 mg q 3–4 hr
4. Determine the dosage ordered
5. Divide the dosage ordered by the maximal recommended dosage to determine their relationship
   Example:
   Drug order: Codeine elixir, 20–30 mg q 3–4 hr
   Maximal dose: 30 mg
   20 mg ordered/30 mg maximum = 66% of therapeutic maximum
   30 mg ordered/30 mg maximum = 100% of therapeutic maximum
The dosage options are between 66% and 100% of the maximal safe dose

---

From Foster R., & Stevens, B. (1994). Nursing management of pain in children. In C. Betz, M. Hunsberger & S. Wright (Eds.), *Family-centered nursing care of children.* Philadelphia: Saunders.

Children should not have to endure pain to achieve pain relief. IM injections are traumatic. Children will quickly learn that it is easier to tolerate pain than report it. The role of the nurse in this situation is to advocate for more appropriate routes of analgesic administration and to educate physicians about age-appropriate pain control strategies.

Intravenous Route

Intravenous (IV) administration is a widely accepted method of delivery in children, but requires monitoring and knowledge about the recommended rate of delivery. IV administration is preferred following surgery and is suitable for titrated bolus or continuous administration.

CASE STUDY

Adrianna, age 4, underwent orthopedic surgery 2 days ago. She is in a full spica cast. Neurovascular assessment is normal. Adrianna is irritable, restless, and is refusing all oral intake. She becomes visibly upset when her 2-year-old sibling visits and screams loudly when her mother attempts to comfort her. The nurse feels that Adrianna is "just upset because her sibling is getting more attention than she is." The mother expresses concern that Adrianna has not rested since the cast application. Adrianna had intramuscular pain medication ordered before surgery; her current orders are for acetaminophen PO every 4 hours prn pain. The nurse offers to give the pain medication to help calm Adrianna down. The nursing priority is to request intravenous medication, either by continuous infusion or intermittent administration every 1 to 3 hours. Adrianna's pain is not being managed with acetaminophen. Adding codeine is not an appropriate alternative at this time because of its slow onset of action and Adrianna's refusal of oral intake. To avoid the "catch-up" phenomenon, pain control will be best achieved with intravenous medications. A pain experience history should have been completed upon admission and reviewed by all health care providers. Once Adrianna's pain is managed appropriately, nonpharmacologic interventions can be identified with input from the child, her parents, the nurse, and the child life specialist.

CASE STUDY

Robert, age 11, has been admitted to the pediatric unit after being struck by an automobile while skateboarding. His injuries include a fractured pelvis, left femur, and left humerus. His anticipated length of stay will be approximately 3 weeks. Since admission, he has consistently rated his pain as 4 on a scale of 0 to 10. He is currently receiving 50 mg Demerol IV every 4 hours prn pain. He requests the pain medication every 1 to 2 hours, but the nurse tells him "he will have to wait, because his medication is not due yet." His physician believes that Robert likes the "rush" he gets with the Demerol® and therefore requests it more frequently. Robert yells loudly every time he is moved and begs his father to do something about the pain. The nurse feels he is not cooperative when laboratory tests or vital signs are due. The nursing priority is to review the pain record and request patient-controlled analgesia (PCA). Robert's pain is inadequately treated due to the peaks and valleys obtained from intermittent prn dosing. His pain rating has not changed since admission, and his behavior is appropriate for someone not achieving optimal pain relief. PCA administration is an excellent alternative at this time. Continuous infusion combined with self-administered bolus dosing will help Robert achieve improved pain control: morphine or hydromorphone should be considered as alternatives to Demerol®. Once Robert's pain is better controlled and his pain ratings decrease, an oral combination therapy of morphine (timed-release) plus a nonopioid agent is recommended.

Patient-Controlled Analgesia

Superior pain relief can be achieved through patient-controlled analgesia (PCA) and can be used safely and effectively in children as young as 3 years of age (Gureno & Reisinger, 1991). PCA is a method of continuous IV administration. The child may also self-administer a small bolus of medication with the use of a hand-operated device. The computerized pump can deliver a bolus dose on demand at intervals determined by the pump's programmer.

PCA is extremely effective for postoperative pain, sickle cell pain, pain caused by tumor encroachment, and pain associated with terminal illness. Even though PCA is recommended for children who possess the cognitive ability to understand the concepts of PCA and the developmental maturity to self-administer bolus doses, parents can take an active role in pain control assistance with PCA administration if the child is not able (Table 11–7).

TABLE 11–7   *PCA Guidelines for Children*

BENEFITS
  Relatively constant plasma concentrations
  Decreased incidence of substantial postoperative
    pain
  Minimal sedation
  Improved mobilization
  Individualized/flexible dosing
  Not a "shot"
  Increased patient/parent control and satisfaction
  Decreased hospital stay
DRUG OPTIONS
  Morphine
  Hydromorphone
  Fentanyl
DOSING GUIDELINES (for postoperative pain)
  Morphine sulfate (approximate dose ranges used:
    actual doses depend on assessment of indi-
    vidual child)
  Loading dose: 0.05–0.20 mg/kg
  PCA dose (bolus): 0.01–0.02 mg/kg
  Lockout interval: usually 5–15 min.
  4-hr limit (optional): 0.30–0.40 mg/kg
  Continuous rate (optional): 0.01–0.04 mg/kg/hr
COMPLICATIONS
  Pump failure or malfunction
  Misprogramming of pump (can result in under-
    medication or overmedication)

Data from: Birmingham, P. (1995). Recent advances in acute pain management. In *Current problems in pediatrics,* (Vol. 25, 3, pp. 92–112). St. Louis, MO: Mosby Yearbook Publishers; Taketomo, C., Hodding, J., & Kraus, D. (1996). *Pediatric dosage handbook* (3rd ed.). Cleveland, OH: Lexi-Comp; Howe, C., Mason, K., & Gordin, P. (1996). Pain and aversive stimuli. In M. Curley, J. Smith, & P. Harmon, *Critical care nursing of infants and children* (pp. 544–547). Philadelphia: Saunders.

Epidural and Intrathecal Administration

Recent advances have made it possible to treat children's pain via epidural and intrathecal routes. A tiny catheter is placed by an anesthesiologist into the epidural or intrathecal space of the spinal column and an opioid is instilled via continuous drip or intermittent administration. Analgesia results primarily from the drug's direct effect on opiate receptors in the spinal cord, rather than in the brain as is true with adults. Compared to traditional intravenous or PCA administration, smaller doses of opiate given via an epidural or intrathecal catheter provide adequate pain control with less sedation (Betz & Sowden, 1996).

Education and competency validation are required for nursing care of the child receiving epidural and intrathecal drug administration. Careful monitoring of catheter placement, oxygen saturation, cardiorespiratory status, potential infection, seizure activity, and patient response are high-priority assessment concerns (Table 11–8).

Topical Administration

Minimizing pain and emotional distress during painful procedures is important in children. One way in which this can be achieved is with the use of topical anesthetics. EMLA® cream (eutectic mixture of local anesthetics) offers a noninvasive method of producing dermal anesthesia in children before the initiation of painful and traumatic nonemergent clinical procedures such as bone marrow aspiration, lumbar puncture, intravenous access, and arterial punctures. Medical centers report its effectiveness with implanted port access, cardiac catheterization preparation, and venipunctures for laboratory tests (Nagenast, 1993). EMLA® cream is applied in a "dollop" or mounded fashion directly from the tube. It is then covered with an occlusive dressing and allowed to sit on the skin for a minimum of 1 hour or as long as 4 hours. The cream is then removed and the procedure is performed.

EMLA® cream is approved for use in children over 1 month of age, but should be used cautiously on

TABLE 11-8   *Epidural Guidelines for Children*

BENEFITS
  Decreased respiratory depression and sedation
  Anesthetic agents can be delivered directly along
    the spinal cord resulting in highly effective pain
    relief
  Improved patient mobility
  Improved analgesia without frequent injections or
    cumbersome I.V. equipment
DRUG OPTIONS*
  Bupivacaine
  Morphine sulfate (preservative free)
  Fentanyl
DOSING GUIDELINES
  Bupivacaine: 0.5 ml/kg of 0.25% (loading dose),
    0.08 ml/kg/hr continuous infusion
  Morphine sulfate: (preservative free) 0.03–0.05
    mg/kg (30–50 µg/kg)
  Fentanyl: dosing guidelines not established; start-
    ing dose usually 10%–20% of IV dose
COMPLICATIONS
  Respiratory depression (early onset 2–4 hr; late
    onset 8–24 hr)
  Urinary retention
  Nausea and vomiting
  Pruritus (especially around face)
  Hypotension
  Sensory and motor blockade
  Catheter migration

Data from Taketomo, C., Hodding, J., & Kraus, D. (1996). *Pediatric
dosage handbook* (3rd ed.). Cleveland, OH: Lexi-Comp; Howe, C.,
Mason, K., & Gordin, P. (1996). Pain and aversive stimuli. In M. Curley,
J. Smith, & P. Harmon, *Critical care nursing of infants and children* (pp.
544–547). Philadelphia: Saunders.
Note:* Meperidine (Demerol) is not recommended for chronic use of
more than 48 hours because of normeperidine toxicity.

infants receiving sulfonamides, phenytoin, or acetaminophen (may increase risk of overt methanoglo-
binemia). Additional precautions include age-appropriate safety guidelines to prevent ingestion of the
cream, removal and ingestion of the occlusive dressing,
and accidental eye exposure. Use of EMLA® cream
appears to decrease the emotional and physical trauma
associated with painful procedures.

Nonpharmacologic Intervention

Numerous nonpharmacologic interventions exist to help children reduce their fear and anxiety and control their pain experience. Child life specialists are especially helpful with these strategies and play an important role in identifying coping mechanisms unique to each child.

Growth and development must be considered when selecting nonpharmacologic interventions for children. General methods include:

- *Infants:* holding, cuddling, sucking a pacifier, massage, soothing music
- *Toddlers:* cuddling, rocking, clutching security object, parent closeness
- *Preschoolers:* engaging in therapeutic play, watching television or a video
- *School-age:* talking about pleasant experiences, playing video games, reading stories
- *Adolescents:* friend and classmate visitation, listening to music, playing video games, sleeping, keeping a journal

Specific strategies for nonpharmacologic pain management include:

- Forming a trusting relationship with the child and family
- Always being honest and truthful
- Staying with the child during a painful procedure
- Educating the family about pain, especially about what to expect
- Involving the family in nonpharmacologic strategies as much as possible
- Avoiding evaluative statements or descriptions of pain (e.g., "this will really hurt a lot")
- Avoiding suggestion of pain; use alternative terms such as "pushing, pinching, or sticking" to describe painful sensations

For long-term pain control, use medical play dolls, and allow the child to treat the doll in the same way he or she is being treated (Table 11–9).

Monitoring the Effectiveness of Pain Control Interventions

When evaluating the effectiveness of pain control interventions, consider the physical and behavioral indicators that lead to the conclusion that pain existed initially. Assessment results should be compared to baseline assessment data. Effective pain management is achieved when (1) the child expresses less pain through verbal, behavioral, and physiologic parameters; (2) the child's goal for pain relief has been met; and (3) the parents estimate the pain as less.

A child's level of pain should be evaluated at regular intervals to determine whether the analgesic reduced, eliminated, or had no affect at all on pain. With effective pain management, a dramatic reduction in pain should occur, although the pain may not disappear completely. Do not misinterpret sleep as an indicator of pain relief. Children will sleep to escape emotional or traumatic situations, and sleep does not necessarily indicate pain control.

Appropriate pain management in children is a collaborative and multidisciplinary effort, in which the physicians, nurses, and parents are key team members. If upon assessment pain interventions are determined inadequate, reassessment and development of a new plan must take place. Consider the drug and its route and frequency of administration, reevaluate the child's pain history, and review other diagnosis-related symptoms that may interfere with pain control measures.

Documentation of pain and pain relief remains one of the most poorly documented parameters nurses assess (Foster & Stevens, 1994). Therefore, a pain assessment record must be used to monitor the effectiveness of all interventions. Several tools are available to document pediatric pain management. At the minimum, pain assessment records should include a pain scale that clearly indicates the intensity of a child's pain, its location, aggravating factors, alleviat-

TABLE 11–9 *Strategies for Nonpharmacologic Pain Management*

DISTRACTION	RELAXATION	GUIDED IMAGERY
Children in severe pain cannot be distracted	Have child assume a comfortable position, or go limp like a rag doll	*This method is most effective for children over 6 years of age*
Involve parent and child in identifying strong distractors	Use progressive relaxation: starting with the toes and systematically let each body part go limp	Have child identify a favorite place, event, or funny story unrelated to the pain process
Use humor, such as watching cartoons, telling jokes or funny stories	Rock in a wide, rhythmic arc, or sway child back and forth, rather than bouncing	Have the child think about the sights, smells, sounds, tastes, and feelings associated with a pleasant experience
Have child blow bubbles to "blow the hurt away"	Have child repeatedly take a deep breath and slowly release it	Combine this method with relaxation
Have child focus on a picture while counting		
Have child listen to music, sing a song, or yell when it hurts		

Adapted from Wong, D. (1995). *Nursing care of infants and children.* St. Louis, MO: Mosby.

ing factors, medications used, sedation scale, and a section to evaluate effectiveness. The pain record should be reviewed on each shift, during patient rounds, and before decisions are made to alter the current plan of care (Figures 11–1 and 11–2).

Patient Education

Children and their families should be actively involved in pain assessment and management. Pain management is optimized when children and parents participate with physicians and nurses in identifying and treating pain (Hester & Foster, 1992). Families should be encouraged to take an active part in assessing, treating, and evaluating their child's pain.

Upon discharge, children are frequently sent home with oral analgesics. Safety precautions must be reviewed to prevent accidental ingestion. Parents should be taught about the dosage, frequency, side effects, and storage of all medications. Parents also should be instructed that a sudden increase in pain intensity may indicate the development of a complication and to seek medical attention at once. Child and parent education is a vital component of the pediatric nurse's role.

Text continued on page 226

Clinical Accountabilities

1. Assess a child's pain not by adult criteria, but by developmental level and previous pain experiences. Assessment of pain can be complex because of constant physical and developmental flux.

2. Look for pain behaviors common to the age group. Remember that children regress developmentally in stressful situations, such as hospitalization.

3. Involve parents in the pain history to learn the child's coping strategies and developmental level. Children's verbal statements and descriptions of pain are the most important factors.

Clinical Accountabilities *(Continued)*

4. Calculate pediatric dosages based on the child's weight in kilograms. Unlike adult dose ranges, pediatric dosages vary individually based on body weight.

5. Do not interpret sleep as an indicator of pain relief. Children will sleep to escape emotionally upsetting or traumatic situations.

6. Avoid IM injections in children.

7. Consider PCA for superior pain control. PCA can be used safely and effectively in children as young as 3 years of age.

8. Value and use nonpharmacologic pain management strategies, especially distraction, relaxation, and guided imagery techniques.
   - Elicit the help of parents to learn these strategies.
   - Ensure they are age-appropriate.

9. Rely on a multidisciplinary and collaborative approach, using the parent and child as key team members. Involving parents helps them regain a sense of control.

10. Monitor the effectiveness of analgesic interventions by comparing current physical and behavioral indicators against baseline data. Completing pain records and documenting pain responses will enable caregivers to customize and/or revise pain control strategies.

11. Recognize pain management as effective when:
    - The child expresses less pain through verbal statements, behavioral cues, and physiologic parameters.
    - The child's goal for pain relief is met.
    - Parents estimate their child's pain as less.

12. Educate the parents about safe storage and administration of medications.
    - Review all discharge medications, and provide the parents with the appropriate resources for follow-up needs.

PEDIATRIC PLAN
OF CARE

Standard #400.01

SYSTEM: General Pediatric
MEDICAL DIAGNOSIS/PROCEDURE: All that apply

NURSING DIAGNOSIS
Pain Related to:

See interdisciplinary problem list for goal statement/evaluations and consultations. See nurses' notes and/or Patient Education Record for all documented interventions and education.

START DATE TIME/INITIALS			DC'D DATE TIME/INITIALS
	ASSESSMENT		
	1. Assess potential for pain (e.g., postoperative, fractures, dressing changes).		
	2. Complete pain experience history record.		

216

3. Use developmentally appropriate scale; have child describe pain by either pointing to faces scale or using 0–5 scale.

4. Assess child for pain characteristics every shift and prn such as:

   a. Location

   b. Type of intensity

   c. Duration

   d. Pattern (constant or intermittent)

   e. Precipitating or aggravating factors

5. Evaluate degree of pain relief after each pain management intervention.

   a. Note changes in pain score, vital signs, behavior.

   b. Question child and/or family regarding satisfaction with pain relief.

6. Assess sleep/rest pattern every shift.

FIGURE 11–1 *Standard of Care for Pediatric Pain* Source: Delgado, V., Kanady, L., & Welsch, E. (1996). *Pediatric pain standard.* Fontana, CA: Kaiser Foundation Hospital Standards of Care.

Illustration continued on following page

Start Date Time/Initials			Dc'd Date Time/Initials
	7. Monitor vital signs and blood pressure per policy and prn.		
	8. Consult child's family on admission concerning child's previous pain experience and response.		
	INTERVENTIONS		
	1. Document assessment, changes in patient's condition, abnormal findings, and interventions/education and effectiveness.		
	2. Provide analgesics as ordered and as needed, and report to physician if child's pain is not effectively relieved.		
	a. Before and after giving IV analgesics, assess level of sedation, respiratory status, and vital signs per policy. (See IV Agreement and special Conditions)		
	b. Notify MD if respiratory rate is decreased and/or child is difficult to arouse.		
	3. Monitor child for side effects of narcotics such as oversedation, itching, urinary retention, constipation, nausea and vomiting, hypotension, and respiratory depression. Notify physician and provide relief measures as ordered.		

218

4. Provide diversional activities as appropriate for age.

a. Music, movies, video games, breathing techniques

5. Maintain family/child contact and encourage family to provide comfort measures.

6. Provide comfort measures such as:

a. Repositioning

b. Warm compress

c. Massage

d. Decreased environmental noise/light

7. Have comfort objects available:

a. Pacifiers, bottle

b. Blankets

c. Favorite toy or stuffed animal from home

FIGURE 11-1 *Continued*

Illustration continued on following page

219

START DATE TIME/INITIALS					DC'D DATE TIME/INITIALS
		8. Touch, comfort, hold child, and use soft voice or music (use reassuring, soft voice at all times). Utilize "baby cuddler" volunteers when available and appropriate.			
		9. Administer analgesics before any painful procedures.			
		10. Encourage appropriate and increasing levels of activity and function.			
		11. Give positive reinforcement for attempts at normal activity patterns (e.g., sitting in a chair, ambulating, self-care activities).			
		12. Encourage use of Child Life Program.			
		13. Explain honestly to child and family when procedures will be painful and expected duration of pain. Avoid pain descriptors.			
		14. If ordered, provide patient-controlled analgesia (PCA) per Hospital Policy to ensure safe and effective pain management.			
		EDUCATION 1. Explain to child and family pain management goals and techniques, including use of analgesics, diversional activity and other comforting measures specific for their child.			

2. Instruct child and family in the safe use of PCA if indicated.								
3. Instruct child and family in the use of pain scale to identify pain level.								
4. Teach family information on alternate methods of pain relief.								
a. Massage								
b. Relaxation exercises								
c. Positioning								
d. Diversional activities/therapeutic play								
5. Give verbal and written instructions to parents on use of analgesics upon discharge.								
a. Effects and side effects								
b. Dosage								
c. Frequency of administration								
d. Safety related to storage and handling								

FIGURE 11-1 *Continued*

Standard #400.19 _____

SYSTEM: General Pediatric
MEDICAL DIAGNOSIS/PROCEDURE: All that apply

NURSING DIAGNOSIS
Chronic pain over six months' duration related
to recurrent or ongoing pathology.

See interdisciplinary problem list for goal statement/evaluations
and consultations. See nurses' notes and/or Patient Education
Record for all documented interventions and education.

Start Date Time/Initials			Dc'd Date Time/Initials
		ASSESSMENT 1. Assess child for pain characteristics every shift and PRN to reduce the likelihood of escalating pain behaviors. Use developmentally appropriate scale, have child describe pain by either pointing to faces scale or using 0–5 scale.	

		DC'D DATE TIME/INITIALS
2. On admission and PRN, obtain pain history/coping mechanism, duration, quality, location and exacerbating and relieving factors including previous pharmacologic trials and any side effects.		
3. Assess effectiveness of pain relief interventions, initiation of treatment, when treatment changes are made, and when patient reports lack of relief.		
INTERVENTIONS 1. Document assessment, changes in patient's condition or pain level, and interventions, including education, and their effectiveness.		
2. Provide analgesics as ordered and as needed, and report to physician if child's pain is not effectively relieved.		
3. Accept child's perception of pain without judgment, realizing behaviors may differ from their rating of pain.		
START DATE TIME/INITIALS		

FIGURE 11–2 *Pediatric Plan of Care Source:* Delgado, V., Kanady, L., & Welsch, E. (1996). *Pediatric pain standard.* Fontana, CA: Kaiser Foundation Hospital Standards of Care.

Illustration continued on following page

Start Date Time/Initials					Dc'd Date Time/Initials			
				4. Monitor child for side effects of narcotics such as: oversedation, constipation, pruritus, rash, nausea and vomiting, respiratory depression, and hypotension. Notify MD of side effects, and provide relief measures as indicated.				
				5. Provide age-appropriate comfort measures such as:				
				a. Physical measures (massage, repositioning, warmth to affected area, touch, comfort, and holding child).				
				b. Distraction (music, movies, video games, use Child Life Program).				
				6. If ordered, provide patient-controlled analgesia (PCA) per Hospital Policy to ensure safe and effective pain management.				
				EDUCATION				
				1. Explain to child and family pain management goals and techniques, including use of analgesics, diversional activity, and other comforting measures specific for their child.				
				2. Instruct child and family on use of PCA pump for hospital and/or home use.				
				3. Teach family information on alternate methods of pain relief.				
				a. Massage				

224

b. Relaxation exercises

c. Positioning

d. Diversional activities/therapeutic play

4. Teach parents symptoms of chronic pain and possible coping behaviors.

5. Give verbal and written instructions to parents on use of analgesics after discharge including:

a. Effects and side effects

b. Dosage

c. Frequency of administration

d. Safety related to storage and handling

FIGURE 11-2 *Continued*

BIBLIOGRAPHY

Acute Pain Management Guideline Panel. (1992). *Acute pain management in infants, children, and adolescents: Operative and medical procedures. Quick reference guide for clinicians.* AHCPR Pub. No. 92-0020. Rockville, MD: Agency for Health Care Policy and Research, Public Health Service, U.S. Department of Health and Human Services.

American Pain Society, Committee on Quality Assurance Standards. (1990). Standards for monitoring quality of analgesic treatment of acute pain and cancer pain. *Oncology Nursing Forum, 17,* 952–954.

Anonymous. (May 1993). *Management of Childhood pain: New approaches to procedure-related pain.* Proceedings of a roundtable discussion. Palm Beach, FL, January 9, 1993. *Journal of Pediatrics, 122*(5 pt 2), S1–46.

Aradine, C.R., Beyer, J.E., & Tompkins, J.M. (1988). Children's pain perception before and after analgesia: A study of instrument construct validity and related issues. *Journal of Pediatric Nursing, 3,* 11–23.

Ball, J., & Bindler, R. (1995). *Pediatric nursing: Caring for children.* East Norwalk, CN: Appleton & Lange.

Berde, C.B. (1989). Pediatric postoperative pain management. *Pediatric Clinics of North America, 36,* 921–940.

Behrman, R., Kliegman, R., Arvin, A., & Nelson, W. (1996). *Textbook of pediatrics* (15th ed., pp. 2058–2078). Philadelphia: Saunders.

Betz, C., & Sowden, L. (1996). *Mosby's pediatric nursing reference.* (3rd Ed.). St. Louis, MO: Mosby.

Birmingham, P. (1995). Recent advances in acute pain management. In *Current problems in pediatrics, vol. 25, 3,* (92–112). St. Louis, MO: Mosby Yearbook Publishers.

Burokas, L. (1985). Factors affecting nurses' decisions to medicate pediatric patients after surgery. *Heart Lung, 14,* 185.

Delgado, V., Kanady, L., Welsch, E. (1996). *Pediatric Pain Standard.* Fontana, CA: Kaiser Foundation Hospital Standards of Care.

Foster, R., & Stevens, B. (1994). Nursing management of pain in children. In C. Betz, M. Hunsberger, & S. Wright (Eds.), *Family-centered nursing care of children* (pp. 882–914). Philadelphia: Saunders.

Gureno, M., & Reisinger, C. (1991). Patient controlled analgesia for the young pediatric patient. *Pediatric Nursing, 17*(3), 251–254.

Hester, N. (1979). The preoperational child's reaction to immunizations. *Nursing Research, 28,* 250–254.

Hester, N. (1993). Pain in children. *Annual Review of Nursing Research, 11,* 105–142.

Hester, N., & Barcus, C. (1986). *Assessment and management of pain in children. Pediatrics: Nursing Update, 1,* 2–8. Princeton, NJ: CPEC, Inc.

Hester, N., & Foster, R. (1992). Children in pain: Research combats undertreatment. *Denver Medical Journal, 1* (2), 20–21.

Howe, C., Mason, K., & Gordin, P. (1996). Pain and aversive stimuli. In M. Curley, J. Smith & P. Harmon, *Critical care nursing of infants and children* (pp. 544–547). Philadelphia: Saunders.

Johnson, K.B. (1993). *The Johns Hopkins Hospital. The Harriet Lane handbook* (13th ed.). St. Louis, MO: Mosby.

Lincoln, L.M. (1992). Children's response to acute pain: A developmental approach. *Journal of the American Academy of Nurse Practitioners, 4*(4), 139–142.

McCaffery, M., & Beebe, A. (1989). *Pain: Clinical manual for nursing practice.* St. Louis: Mosby.

McGrath, P.J., & McAlpine, L. (1993). Psychologic perspectives on pediatric pain. *Journal of Pediatrics, 122* (5 pt 2), S2–8.

Nagenast, S. (1993). The use of EMLA® cream to reduce and/or eliminate procedural pain in children. *Journal of Pediatric Nursing, 8*(6), 406–407.

Nelson, W., Behrman, R., Kliegman, R., & Arvin, A. (1996). *Textbook of pediatrics* (15th ed.). Philadelphia: Saunders.

Pfefferbaum, B., & Hagberg, C.A. (1993). Pharmacological management of pain in children. *Journal of the American Academy of Child and Adolescent Psychiatry, 32*(2), 235–242.

Savedra, M., Holzemer, W., & Ward, J. (1989). *Adolescent pediatric pain tool (APPT): Preliminary user's manual.* San Francisco: University of California.

Stevens, B., Johnston, C.C. (1993). Pain in the infant: Theoretical and conceptual issues. *Maternal-Child Nursing Journal, 21*(1), 3–14.

Steward, M.D., & O'Connor, J. (1994). Pediatric pain, trauma and memory. *Current Opinion in Pediatrics, 6*(4), 411–417.

Taketomo, C., Hodding, J., & Kraus, D. (1996). *Pediatric dosage handbook* (3rd ed.). Cleveland, OH: Lexi-Comp.

Vessey, J.A., Carlson, K.L., & McGill, J. (1994). Use of

distraction with children during an acute pain experience. *Nursing Research, 43*(6), 369–372.

Walco, G.A., Cassidy, R.C., & Schechter, N.L. (1994). Pain, hurt, and harm. The ethics of pain control in infants and children. *New England Journal of Medicine, 331*(8), 541–544.

Wong, D. (1995). *Nursing care of infants and children.* St. Louis, MO: Mosby.

Wong, D., & Whaley, L. (1986). *Clinical handbook of pediatric nursing* (2nd ed., p. 373). St. Louis, MO: Mosby.

12
Pain in the Older Adult

Although since the mid-1980s more attention has been paid to the needs and care of the elderly, research about pain management and the geriatric population is still limited. Pain is a significant problem among the elderly as a symptom of disease and because it entails more frequent use of the health care system. Estimates indicate that from 25% to 50% of older adults in the community suffer from pain (Crook et al, 1984); and the percentage increases to as high as 80% in long-term care facilities (Ferrell et al., 1990). Pain impacts the elderly in a variety of ways, including decreased quality of life, impaired functional abilities, diminished social activities, reduced cognitive status, altered nutritional state, and sleep difficulties (Roche & Forman, 1994). Pain in the elderly is associated with increased use of health care services, which generate higher costs to the health care system and to the older adult health care consumer. In addition, older adults present with unique pain management problems because of concomitant chronic illnesses, alterations in pain reporting and pain assessment, and associated risks entailed in using analgesic medications.

PAIN INCIDENCE AND PERCEPTIONS

What is Pain to the Older Adult?

Pain is the feeling of being hurt, the awareness of suffering discomfort, and is the most common reason people seek health care. Pain is a common companion of the frail elderly that overemphasizes the negatives of normal aging. It clouds thinking and slows movement. Pain can so cleverly disguise itself as part of the normal aging process that pain-impaired seniors may not seek relief.

Epidemiology

Pain is prevalent among the elderly. Some studies estimate that 80% to 85% of adults over the age of 65 years have at least one major health problem that may predispose them to pain (Harkins, 1988). The painful diseases that are most common among the elderly include arthritis and cancer. Arthritis may occur in 80% of those over 65 years, and most of those with this disease will suffer some degree of pain. Among cancer patients, one-third of those undergoing active treatment and two-thirds of those with advanced disease experience severe pain. Other painful conditions that occur more often among older adults than the younger population include temporal arteritis, polymyalgia rheumatica, herpes zoster, osteoporosis, vertebral compression fractures, falls, and peripheral vascular disease.

Is Pain Perceived Differently in the Elderly?

The perception of pain is a highly individual process specific to each older adult. Generalizations regarding age-related pain sensitivity are difficult to document. Some studies report decreases in pain perception in the elderly (Enck, 1991), whereas others show no change in sensitivity to pain with age (Harkins, 1988). Age does not appear significantly to affect the sensory dimensions of pain in the "well elderly" (Harkins, 1988). However, controlled experimental laboratory studies do not take into account the effects of cultural and psychosocial factors that may influence pain perception. Likewise, induced pain studies do not necessarily stimulate recurrent or chronic pains or the clinical situation in which pain is experienced. Therefore, it must be concluded that pain perception is a highly complex process that depends on a multitude of internal and external factors. Pain perception cannot be generalized among the older adult population;

rather, individualized perceptions and reports of pain must be acknowledged by health care providers.

Pain Beliefs

Some beliefs among both the elderly and health care providers have an impact on both assessment and pain management strategies. Recognizing these beliefs is crucial to the development of a comprehensive plan for relieving pain. Ignoring them can be detrimental to the care of older adults who are in pain.

Clinically, the presence and degree of pain are most accurately determined by the person who is hurting, not by the caregiver. Older adults often present as "good patients." They may fear to express complaints of pain because such complaints may affect quality of care. A desire to "please the doctor" is a common reason why seniors often limit their reporting. Steele (1992) has shown that physicians may spend *less* time with patients whose pain has *not* responded to treatment. Furthermore, family members may reinforce the "good patient" role if the older relative does not "complain too much." Elders themselves often choose not to make their pain known for fear of "becoming a burden" to their families.

Older adults may not report pain either because they fear tests, operations, and/or treatment costs. An older adult who has had a painful experience during an MRI or CAT scan where there was a need to stay still for some time, may opt to minimize reporting arthritic pain because the test appears to be more important than the chronic pain.

Finally, many seniors believe that reporting pain will result in the use of addicting drugs that symbolize the end of independent functioning. If opioids are prescribed, the elderly may perceive that death is imminent, sustaining the belief that potent pain killers are reserved for the dying. If the older adult has previously taken a medication with a sedative effect, there may be an associated fear that stronger pain medications may diminish mental function and/or ability to perform activities of daily living.

It is important to explore the older adult's beliefs and previous experiences with pain management to avoid the underreporting of pain. Health care professionals need to explain the benefits and side effects of medications, as well as the risk of psychologic and physical dependence. Each fear or belief must be recognized and addressed, so that the health care professional can allay the fear and optimally educate the patient. The patient and family must be included in the development of the pain management plan whenever possible.

Pain perception in the elderly also is affected by the beliefs of health care professionals. Pain should not be accepted simply as a normal part of aging. Physiologically, aging does not cause pain. Pain is a signal of disease or impending dysfunction. However, chronic illnesses do cause pain, and many elderly people have at least one chronic illness. Many health professionals continue to view some pain in the elderly as "normal." Perhaps this explains in part why pain is often undertreated in the elderly.

Another belief that many health care professionals hold is that pain often is psychogenic in the older adult. In fact, pain may be associated with anxiety and depression, but pain resulting purely from a psychological origin is unusual in the elderly.

Some health care professionals are hesitant to provide adequate doses of opioids to older adults for fear of promoting respiratory depression or psychologic dependence (addiction). This may be another reason for undertreatment of pain in the elderly. In fact, the most common adverse side effects associated with opioid analgesic use in the elderly are constipation and confusion. Psychologic dependence on opioids is rare in the older adult and respiratory depression uncommon. The dosage of opioids should be individualized for every patient and based on need, effectiveness, and evidence of side effects.

ASSESSMENT: SPECIAL CHALLENGES

Older adults require comprehensive pain assessment for several reasons. Pain is the most common symptom of disease and proper assessment is necessary for accurate diagnosis and treatment of the disease process. Adequacy of pain relief must be evaluated by ongoing individual patient reassessment. Without reassessment, older adults are at risk for undertreatment or, less commonly, overtreatment of pain. Lastly, comprehensive pain assessment provides the comparative data necessary for distinguishing a new disease process from existing chronic conditions (Ferrell & Ferrell, 1990).

Accurately identifying pain in an older adult can be difficult. Frail elders often present with multiple vague and overlapping symptoms that are difficult to evaluate. Angina pectoris, for instance, may be described as diffuse abdominal pain plus shortness of breath. Severe hip pain often presents as a simple refusal to ambulate associated with a loss of appetite. Although a careful history and physical examination, plus focused lab and x-ray testing, will facilitate accurate pain assessment, an observed decrease in "usual function" is, perhaps, the most sensitive indicator of pain in the frail older adult. This variable becomes even more important for older adults who are unable to comprehend and use pain assessment tools. Pain may have an impact on participation in recreational activities or social events. Walking, transferring, and posture may be impaired. Pain-related sleep disturbances, depression, and anxiety may be experienced. Poor appetite and constipation may also develop, as well as incontinence and impaired memory and grooming.

During the assessment, the patient should be observed for any overt behaviors, including guarding, facial grimaces, and agitated behavior. It must be remembered, however, that patients in pain may not exhibit any outward signs of discomfort. The only visible sign may be slowness of movement, which may be mistaken for a normal part of the aging process.

Comprehensive pain assessment includes a detailed history and physical examination. The physical examination should include palpation for any trigger points or areas of inflammation. Trigger points may be caused by tendinitis, muscle strain, or nerve irritation. The neurologic examination may reveal deficits indicative of neuropathic syndromes or nerve damage. Selected laboratory tests, including a complete blood count and sedimentation rate, may indicate infection, polymyalgia rheumatica, or temporal arteritis. A high uric acid level may correlate with suspected gout.

Those with chronic pain may be aided by a psychologic evaluation for depression and anxiety, problems that might benefit from treatment. An interdisciplinary approach that includes the patient/family unit is most beneficial.

Pain assessment in the elderly can be complex and will be more reliable when it is performed in the most patient-sensitive manner. For example, is the patient in a comfortable chair or position? Is the room too hot or too cold? Any measures that demonstrate accommodation to the patient as well as a caring attitude will generally be appreciated, allowing the older patient to cooperate more willingly with the assessment process.

Once pain has been identified, it must be quantified to judge treatment efficacy. Many pain measurement tools offer a means for the patient to describe and rate the pain. Visual analog scales with bright red or orange vertical lines are easier for those with decreased visual acuity. Pain diaries may be helpful in correlating what aggravates the pain, what relieves the pain, what coexists with the pain, and how the pain management plan is proceeding. In the cognitively intact individual, a simple 0 to 10 numeric scale will provide adequate quantification of pain.

Acute Pain

Among the elderly, there are variations of expected presentations of acute pain. Older adults may present with painless acute myocardial injury, mesenteric infarction, or appendicitis. In younger adults, this acute pain often is a key symptom for diagnosis. However, in older adults acute pain often is an atypical or referred pain. Health care providers must be vigilant in the absence of expected pain or in the presence of atypical pain presentations. Also, there may be variations in acute pain presentation among the "well elderly" in contrast to the chronically debilitated elderly. Management of acute pain in the elderly is similar to younger adults, but takes into account coexisting chronic conditions, medication interactions, and potential side effects of pharmacologic interventions.

Chronic Pain

Chronic pain most often is associated in the elderly with osteoarthritis and cancer. Chronic pain is devastating among older adults because it reduces functional status. In addition, there often is associated emotional distress and depression.

Dementia and Delirium

Dementia is a chronic irreversible decrease in cognitive function. Delirium is an acute reversible confusion. Patients with dementia are awake and alert, whereas delirious individuals exhibit fluctuating levels of consciousness. Delirium and dementia often impair an elderly patient's ability to communicate pain.

Since the confused older adult may not be able to adequately describe painful sensation, the health care professional must be astute at recognizing behavioral indicators of pain. To make an accurate assessment, the health care professional must be aware of what is "normal" behavior and what is "abnormal" behavior for the individual. For example, Marzinski (1991) found that someone who normally moans and rocks may become withdrawn and quiet when in pain. Another patient with disjointed verbal efforts may momentarily be able to describe the pain location exactly. Someone who is quiet and nonverbal may blink rapidly with hardly noticeable facial grimaces as a pain expression. When hurting, the friendly, outgoing long-term care resident may become agitated and combative, whereas another individual who normally participates in recreational activities may cry easily and withdraw from social interactions. In the confused elder, health care professionals must be acutely aware that pain may be a factor in any observed behavior change.

CASE STUDY

Mrs. B is a 72-year-old female who lives alone in her own home. She is functionally independent in all of her activities of daily living. She drives, does her own shopping, and participates in "Senior Aerobics" twice a week. She self-medicates with over-the-counter NSAIDs for her osteoarthritis and alternates between hot and cold packs for her knees, depending on her activity level and pain sensation.

On her way back from the mailbox, Mrs. B slips and falls on a patch of ice. A neighbor observes the incident and calls 911. Mrs. B is taken to the local hospital where an x-ray confirms a left hip fracture. Mrs. B is taken to surgery. Postoperatively, she is confused and is restrained to maintain hip precautions. She does not report any pain, but tries to remove the restraints. Her nurses assess that the confusion may be secondary to pain and provide the ordered opioid analgesic on a regularly scheduled basis around-the-clock for the first 24 hours.

By the next day, Mrs. B is alert and oriented and is able to utilize a pain scale for reporting pain level and response to analgesic. However, she does not ask for any pain medication because she does not want to "bother the nurse." A float nurse is assigned to her, and this nurse does not offer the opioid because Mrs. B "does not look like she is in pain." This nurse is concerned about oversedation and respiratory depression.

That night Mrs. B again becomes confused and is labeled a "sun-downer." In the morning, she refuses to eat breakfast, and her day nurse inquires about Mrs. B's sleepless, restless night. She is told by Mrs. B that her hip pain is 9 out of 10 and that her knees are 10 out of 10. The day nurse immediately provides the opioid analgesic and requests an order for an nonsteroidal anti-inflammatory drug (NSAID) to be offered with food per Mrs. B's home schedule prior to hospitalization.

In physical therapy, Mrs. B's daughter requests cold pack treatments for her mother's knees after exercises, as this was her treatment method at home. The physical therapist agrees to this adjunct treatment.

By day four, Mrs. B is consistently alert and oriented, is consuming 75% to 100% of her meals, and is progressing with physical therapy. She is taking NSAIDs on a regularly scheduled basis and requests opioid analgesics 1 hour prior to physical therapy and when her self-assessed pain level is rated to be a 6 on a scale of 0 to 10.

Mrs. B is discharged home on scheduled anti-inflammatory medication and a mild opioid analgesic to be used as needed for pain.

KEY POINT

Confusion may be an indication of pain.

Management Issues

There are two core principles in managing pain in older adults: (1) maximize relief; and (2) improve function. Achieving optimal balance between these requisites is challenging. Relief can be defined as reducing or freeing from pain. Function can be defined as the ability to carry out one's activities of daily living. In older adults, attention to only relieving pain *may not* always improve an individual's ability to function in his or her usual way.

For instance, prescribing acetaminophen with codeine for an elder's chronic back pain, may lessen his symptom while causing severe constipation, clouded judgment, and falling. Treating postoperative pain with PRN doses of meperidine and hydroxyzine may intermittently reduce discomfort, but contribute to the development of delirium, use of physical restraints, and increased hospital stay.

Balancing relief with function in an older adult requires a more holistic approach. Humans suffer discomfort in four basic ways: (1) physically; (2) emotionally; (3) socially; and (4) spiritually. As aging tends to result in a certain level of physical discomfort, maintaining "normal function" in old age largely depends on emotional, social, and spiritual adaptations.

Any significant change in a patient's basic or instrumental activities of daily living should prompt a comprehensive search for pain:

Basic activities of daily living

- Toileting
- Dressing
- Bathing
- Feeding
- Mobility
- Continence

Instrumental activities of daily living

- Cooking
- Cleaning
- Washing clothes
- Shopping
- Driving
- Using telephone
- Handling finances

Advanced activities of daily living

- Self-esteem issues
- Future plans
- Recreational preferences and plans

Physical pain tends to impair activities of daily living, whereas emotional, social, and spiritual discomfort tend to present as declines in the instrumental or advanced activities of daily living. Without adequate functional assessment, pain in the elderly will be overlooked and, therefore, undertreated.

TREATMENT CONSIDERATIONS

Comprehensive pain relief in the older adult is based on the application of specific remedies to each component of the pain experience. Treatment focuses on relieving not only the physical but also the emotional, social, and spiritual components of an individual's pain. Treatment modalities can be pharmacologic and nonpharmacologic. Severe pain, especially if chronic, requires the involvement of a multidisciplinary team.

There are some general principles of pain management in the elderly. First of all, each older adult is a highly unique individual. Making generalizations about people and/or pain syndromes is a deterrent in treating elders in pain. There are differences among all individuals, especially among the "well elderly" in contrast to the "frail elderly."

Second, it is necessary to be realistic, forthright, caring and honest in approaching an elder in pain. If a senior citizen wants to have her arthritic knee treated so that she can continue ice skating with her granddaughter, the health care professional must be prepared to work with her to meet those expectations as much as possible.

Third, seniors usually have a past experience of "tried-and-true" remedies for pain relief. Health care professionals need to find out what has worked for the individual in the past. The patient's own observations and judgments about the causes of pain and possible relief measures should be trusted.

Last, time must be allowed for patient education, whether in the form of handouts, videos, simulations, practice sessions, or other methods the patient may prefer. The educational process should be flexible. It should allow for personal interactions, questions and answers, and exploration of concerns and feelings pertaining to the physical, emotional, social, and spiritual aspect of pain.

Pharmacologic Remedies

In general, therapeutic use of analgesics is not impaired by normal aging. However, problems may develop if medications are not administered and monitored appropriately. The aging process itself may put the elderly at risk for analgesic toxicity. Decreased renal function, altered hepatic function, less lean body mass, a longer half-life, as well as slower gastric emptying predispose the elderly to potential adverse effects of some analgesics. Coexisting chronic disease states may also increase the potential for adverse effects. Preexisting kidney or liver disease, congestive heart failure, hypoalbuminemia, or hypoventilation can all contribute to slower metabolism of analgesics, increasing their potential for producing harmful side effects. Interactions with other medications may also influence analgesic toxicities.

Table 12–1 illustrates a simplified approach to the use of analgesic medications in the elderly. Regardless of the drugs utilized, general principles of analgesic pharmacotherapy can be applied:

- Always believe the patient as to the severity of the pain.
- Choose the analgesic most likely to relieve the pain *and* maintain or improve normal functioning.
- *Prevent* the recurrence of pain. Administer analgesic medication on a scheduled basis whenever possible.
- Individualize therapy and reassess at regular intervals.
- Recognize that psychologic dependence is rare.

Nonopioid analgesics, acetaminophen and nonsteroidal anti-inflammatory drugs (NSAIDs) have been used to provide relatively safe and effective relief of mild to moderate pain for many elderly patients. The increased use of NSAIDs in the elderly has provided recognition of significant toxicities and risk factors. Fortunately, many of the associated toxicities can be avoided through a thorough comprehensive approach to pain management.

Gastrointestinal (GI) side effects are most common with the NSAIDs. These discomforts range from

TABLE 12-1 *Analgesic Medication in the Elderly*

Pain Severity Scale	If Acute Pain	If Chronic Pain
1–2 (minimal)	Oral acetaminophen or NSAIDs *as needed** Consider topical analgesics†	Same; may schedule medication use for certain hours of day; i.e., always at bedtime
3–4 (mild)	Oral acetaminophen/NSAID, or oral opioid analgesic.‡ Consider topical analgesics†	Same; may schedule medication throughout waking hours; add disease-specific treatment§
5–7 (moderate)	Parenteral or oral opioid analgesic on scheduled basis (not PRN); may add benzodiazepine anxiolytic for rest or sleep as needed	Oral opioid analgesic on scheduled basis; may add tricyclic antidepressant, and/or oral narcotic analgesic PRN for breakthrough pain, and/or disease specific treatment§
8–10 (severe)	Parenteral opioid analgesic on scheduled basis (not PRN); may add benzodiazepine anxiolytic on scheduled basis	Parenteral or oral opioid analgesic on scheduled basis plus parenteral or oral opioid PRN for break-through pain; plus tricyclic antidepressant; plus disease specific treatment. May add benzodiazepine anxiolytic for rest or sleep

*Use analgesic doses of NSAIDs. Limit total daily dose of acetaminophen to 4 gr per 24 hours.

†Topical salicylate cream or capsaicin creme.

‡Propoxyphene is reported to be no more effective than aspirin or acetaminophen. May use anti-inflammatory doses of NSAIDs.

§Disease-specific analgesic medication may include anticonvulsants for neuropathic pain (Tegretol®, Dilantin®, Klonopin®, Depakote®); corticosteroids for polymyalgia rheumatica; methotrexate for rheumatoid arthritis, etc.

nausea and heartburn to ulceration and bleeding. To minimize these effects, the NSAIDs should be ingested with food. Histamine antagonists may be necessary if GI symptoms are not controlled with food.

Renal toxicity usually is reversible if the patient is monitored for renal insufficiency, hypernatremia, fluid retention, and hyperkalemia. Other side effects are potential bleeding (due to alterations in platelet aggregation), anxiety, dizziness, tinnitus, drowsiness, confusion, bronchospasm, urticaria, and pruritus. Acetaminophen may be the drug of choice if the individual is at risk for bleeding.

Opioids are excellent analgesics but may cause various side effects among the elderly. Older adults are more sensitive to the analgesic effects of opioids and may benefit from smaller doses than younger adults. The elderly may experience constipation and alterations in cognition and respiratory depression with opioid use. In addition, opioids may predispose some older adults to severe agitation. Respiratory depression and psychologic dependence are rare complications of monitored opioid use in the elderly. Withholding opioid analgesics from the older adult because of fear of these complications is unfounded.

The opioids may also trigger nausea and vomiting. In younger patients, nausea and vomiting often are treated with antihistamines and phenothiazines. In the elderly, these antiemetics may themselves produce anticholinergic effects, delirium, and mobility dysfunction. Therefore, avoidance of opioid-related side effects is important. Scheduled dosing of opioids, rather than as-needed dosing may prevent severe nausea and vomiting because tolerance to side effects occurs more quickly than tolerance to analgesia (Ferrell & Ferrell, 1991).

There are a number of drugs of choice for treating pain-associated depression and anxiety in the elderly:

1. *Tricyclic antidepressants*
   a. Norpramine (Desipramine®)
   b. Nortriptyline (Pamelor®)
   c. Amitriptyline (Elavil®); low dose only

2. *Anxiolytic agents*
   a. Lorazepam (Ativan®)
   b. Oxazepam (Serax®)

Depression is most commonly associated with pain lasting more than 3 months (Ferrell, 1991). Anxiety can occur with both acute and chronic discomfort. Amitriptyline, although effective as adjunctive pain treatment, should be avoided because of its excessive adverse side effect profile. Only short-acting benzodiazepine anxiolytics are recommended for use in the elderly. The newer and safer antidepressants (selective serotonin reuptake inhibitors, Wellbutrin®, Serazone®, etc.) are highly effective in reducing depression in the older adult; however, they appear less effective in reducing chronic pain than the more traditional tricyclic antidepressants listed.

Nonpharmacologic Remedies

Pain also can be lessened or relieved by therapies other than medications. Other common nonpharmacologic remedies for relieving physical pain include:

- Transcutaneous electrical nerve stimulation (TENS)
- Physical therapy
- Massage
- Heat or cold application
- Splints or positioning modalities
- Accupuncture/accupressure
- Chiropractic consultation
- Nontraditional exercise programs

Transcutaneous electrical nerve stimulation, along with acupuncture and acupressure, have been shown to relieve pain associated with spinal back injury, diabetic peripheral neuropathy, phantom limb pain, neuralgia, and arthritis (Thomas, 1990). Unfortunately, the relief experienced by these methods may be short-lived (weeks to a few months).

Physical and occupational therapists can provide all sorts of practical help in reducing physical pain in the elderly. Canes, walkers, and splints can relieve pressure on an arthritic or contractured limb, thereby lessening pain. Strengthening or stretching muscles, applying heat or cold, and using local massage also are effective pain-reducing modalities. Consideration of chiropractic manipulation therapy and nontraditional exercise programs such as T'ai Chi may provide still further means of lessening or reducing physical pain in a hurting senior.

A comprehensive, holistic approach also must include treatment of the emotional component of pain. Every human discomfort is associated with some type of emotional response. A partial listing of nondrug treatments that may facilitate positive emotional adjustments in the older adult with pain includes:

- Psychotherapy
- Counseling
- Hypnosis
- Relaxation training
- Guided imagery
- Biofeedback
- Distraction
- Meditation
- Music therapy
- Prayer

Although compliance is difficult to obtain, older adults that do seek emotional support and education seem to hurt less (Thomas, 1990). An elder in pain usually has some type of social support system, most often a family. Adequate pain control depends, in part, on the understanding and expectations of this family. If the caregiving family understands the senior's illness and treatment and believes that the patient is well cared for, they can easily direct the majority of their supportive energy toward their loved one. Patients recognize this energy as encouragement and are better able to cope with their pain. On the other hand, if the patient's family feels uninformed and disconnected from the healing process, the older patient may receive inadequate encouragement, leading to loneliness, depression, and more discomfort.

The family must be kept informed of every aspect of the pain treatment process. The health care professional must ensure that family and patient expectations of treatment outcomes are consistent with the known clinical realities. Connecting the patient–family unit as closely as possible results in shared suffering and lessened pain.

Finally, human spirit can be defined as an individual's most valued reason for living. Severe or prolonged pain has the capacity of clouding over this "core value," leading to apathy. Apathy impairs mental, physical, and emotional concentration, thereby accentuating pain.

One of the best ways to lessen pain is to feed an individual's core reason for living. This can be accomplished by simply showing, in as many ways as possible, that the health care worker genuinely cares for the elder in pain. Giving the senior "worth" will reduce apathy and lessen the perception of pain.

Reevaluation

Once treatment is in progress, ongoing reassessment of pain management is crucial for lasting relief. Is the pain adequately relieved in the mind of both patient and family? Are any adjustments in care needed to better meet patient and family expectations in view of the current clinical realities? Do patient and family fully understand the pain management process?

Pain management in the elderly requires meticulous attention to all the components of suffering—physical discomfort, emotional anguish, social isolation, and spiritual apathy. Only when each of these elements is compassionately assessed and properly managed can optimal pain management be achieved.

Clinical Accountabilities

1. Understand that pain in the elderly is a signal of disease or impending dysfunction; pain is not a normal part of aging.

2. Be alert to the underreporting of pain, to the "good patient" presentation, or fear of "becoming a burden" to one's family.

3. Assess and reassess the older adult comprehensively.
   - Pursue decreased function, slowness of movement as a sign of pain (most sensitive indicator of pain in the frail older adult, especially those who are unable to comprehend or use assessment tools).
   - Be vigilant in assessing for acute pain—often presents in the older adult as atypical or referred pain.
   - Distinguish between dementia and delirium; search for subtle signs of behavior that is "abnormal" for that individual patient (suggests pain).
   - Watch for any behavior change in the confused elder (pain may be a factor).

4. Respect the patient's past experience of "tried-and-true" remedies for pain relief.

5. Maximize relief, and improve function through pharmacologic and nonpharmacologic means.

6. Manage opioid therapy knowledgably.
   - Recognize that with monitored opioid therapy, addiction and respiratory depression are uncommon in the older adult (adequate doses should be administered).
   - Be prepared to counteract the most common side effects of opioids: constipation and confusion.

7. Maximize pain relief and function.
   - Respect the older adult's expectations, and support them to the extent possible, assuring expectations are consistent with clinical realities.

Clinical Accountabilities (Continued)

- Treat individually; differentiate between "well elderly" and "frail elderly."
8. Treat anxiety or depression (commonly associated with chronic pain).
9. Connect the patient/family unit as closely as possible.
10. Look for ways the older adult may contribute to the family, others, or their own sense of self. Give the older adult "worth."

BIBLIOGRAPHY

Acute Pain Management Guideline Panel. (1992). *Acute Pain Management: Operative or Medical Procedures and Trauma.* AHCPR Pub. No. 92–0032. Rockville, MD: U.S. Dept. of Health & Human Services, Agency for Health Care Policy and Research.

Crook, J., Rideout, C., & Brown, G. (1984). The prevalence of pain complaints among a general population. *Pain, 18,* 299–314.

Enck, R.E. (1991). Pain control in the ambulatory elderly. *Geriatrics, 46,* 49–60.

Ferrell, B.A. (1991). Pain management in elderly people. *Journal of American Geriatric Society, 39,* 64–73.

Ferrell, B.A., Ferrell, B.R. (1991). Principles of pain management in older people. *Comprehensive Therapy, 17,* 53–58.

Ferrell, B.A., Ferrell, B.R., & Osterweil, D. (1990). Pain in the nursing home. *Journal of American Geriatrics Society,* 38, 409–414.

Harkins, S.W. (1988). Pain in the elder. In R. Dubner, F.G. Bebhart, & M.D. Bond (Ed.), *Proceedings of the Fifth World Congress on Pain.* Amsterdam: Elsevier, 355–357.

Harkins, S.W., Kwentus, J. & Price, D.D. (1984). Pain in the elderly. In C. Benedetti (Ed.), *Advances in pain research and therapy* (Vol. 7). New York: Raven, 103–212.

Marzinski, L.R. (1991). The tragedy of dementia: Clinically assessing pain in the confused nonverbal elderly. *Journal of Gerontological Nursing, 17,* 6, 25–28.

Roche, J.R., & Forman, W.B. (1994). Pain management for the geriatric patient. *Clinics in Podiatric Medicine and Surgery, 11,* 1, 41–53.

Shahady, E.J. (1990). Difficult patients uncovering the real problems of "crocks" and "gamers." *Consultant,* vol. 24, 33–37, 41–43.

Steele, J.A. (1992). Cancer pain in the elderly needs special attention. *Journal of the National Cancer Institute, 84,* (15), 1153.

Thomas, B.L. (1990). Pain management for the elderly: Alternative interventions (Part I). *AORN, 52,* 1268–1272.

Tucker, M.A., Andrew, M.F., Ogle, S.J., et al. (1989). Age associated change in pain threshold measured by transcutaneous electrical neuronal stimulation. *Age and Aging, 18,* 241–246.

13

Substance Abuse: Assessment and Treatment Challenges

As Payne pointed out, "There are few clinical situations more challenging, frustrating, or stressful than the management of acute or chronic pain in patients known or suspected to be abusers of narcotics or other prescription drugs, alcohol, or illegal substances" (1989, p. 46). As pain management principles rely on the patient's perception of the experience and ability to take control of their situation, the additional challenge of **substance use disorder (SUD)** can make effective pain management quite complex. What is the probability of such presentations? An estimated 15.3 million Americans exhibit symptoms of alcoholism or alcohol dependence (NIAAA, 1993), and 14.5 million Americans currently use illicit drugs (NIDA, 1991). Varied studies have documented the presence of SUD in hospitalized individuals (Fleming & Barry, 1992; Moore, et al, 1989; Reyna, et al, 1985). Substance dependency among nonmalignant pain patients has been estimated at 3.2% to 18.9% (Sees & Clark, 1992). Given the prevalence of pain and of substance use disorders, it is highly likely that clinicians will be faced with providing pain relief to individuals with the dual diagnosis of pain and SUD.

Attitudes and deficiencies in basic knowledge regarding pain assessment and treatment as well as lack of knowledge of SUDs contribute to the challenge. Previous chapters have discussed the principles of pain assessment and treatment; these principles are no different when caring for an individual diagnosed

249

with SUD. In addition to these generic principles, health care professionals need to be familiar with diagnostic criteria for SUD; substance use assessment and screening tools; signs and symptoms of substance-specific intoxication and withdrawal, time course and treatment strategies; and pain treatment strategies employed within the context of SUD.

SUBSTANCE-RELATED DISORDERS

Substance-related disorders are divided into two groups: **substance use disorders** (dependence and abuse) and **substance-induced disorders** (substance-induced intoxication, withdrawal, delirium, persisting dementia, persisting amnesiac disorder, psychotic disorder, mood disorder, anxiety disorder, sexual dysfunction, sleep disorder) (American Psychiatric Association, 1994). **Substance dependence** and **substance abuse** are characterized by maladaptive patterns of substance use that result in clinically significant impairment or distress. The diagnostic criteria for substance use disorders and substance-induced disorders, specifically withdrawal and intoxication, are presented in Table 13–1. The substance-induced disorders, such as delirium and persisting dementia, vary with the substance and exceed the limits of this discussion.

Patients chronically maintained on opioids for pain relief meet several criteria for substance dependence (e.g., **tolerance,** withdrawal, taking larger amounts over a longer period of time than intended, inordinate amount of time spent to obtain substance), yet these individuals would be *inappropriately* diagnosed as substance dependent (Wesson, et al, 1993). Individuals who derive pain relief from opioids typically experience improved function and are able to control use, whereas individuals with SUD are unable to control their use, desire a mood-altering effect rather than pain relief, and continue to use the substance(s) despite harmful or negative consequences.

Likewise, individuals who receive inadequate pain treatment may be inappropriately labeled as substance dependent. The term **pseudoaddiction** describes an iatrogenic syndrome of abnormal behavior developing as a direct consequence of inadequate pain management (Weissman & Haddox, 1986). Pseudoaddiction is manifested by behaviors that mimic dependency, namely an overwhelming and compulsive interest in obtaining and using opioid medications. Requests for more frequent medications, requests for specific medications that have worked in the past, and behaviors that attempt to convince the health care professional of the presence and severity of the pain (e.g., moaning, crying, grimacing, holding affected body parts) may be pseudoaddiction behaviors driven by attempts to seek pain relief. These behaviors may develop in individuals receiving medications on an as-needed basis rather than around-the-clock when pain is continuous and in individuals who are prescribed analgesics with inadequate potency and/or receiving analgesics at intervals that exceed the analgesic activity of the medication.

KEY POINT

The criteria for substance use disorders must be applied within the context of use.

The SUD patient demonstrates a constellation of behaviors that underline the nature of the disorder. It is important to recognize that substance use may be driven by the basic desire to achieve homeostasis, a response to psychologic suffering. Drug taking provides the means to get control by changing one's mood. To illustrate, a heightened awareness of feelings may predispose an individual to use central nervous system (CNS) depressants in order to tone down feelings, or an individual with a sense of blunted feelings may use CNS stimulants to heighten feelings (McCaffery & Vourakis, 1992). Dysphoric mood states, availability of substance, and expectancies of mood alteration or relief of psychologic suffering may be more important than craving or avoidance of physical withdrawal in compulsive substance use (Fleming & Barry, 1992).

TABLE 13–1 *Substance-Related Disorders*

Substance Dependence	Substance Abuse	Substance Intoxication	Substance Withdrawal
Maladaptive pattern of use leading to clinically significant impairment or distress; manifested by 3 or more of the following occurring at any time in a 12-month period:	Maladaptive pattern of use leading to clinically significant impairment or distress; manifested by 1 or more of the following occurring at any time in a 12-month period:	1. Development of reversible substance-specific syndrome due to recent substance use	1. Development of a substance-specific syndrome due to the cessation of or reduction in heavy and prolonged use
1. Tolerance Need for markedly increased amounts of substance to achieve intoxication or desired effect or Markedly diminished effect with continued use of same amount Degree to which tolerance develops on the substance	Criteria for substance abuse do not include tolerance, withdrawal, or a pattern of compulsive use Criteria focus on harmful consequences of repeated substance use	2. Clinically significant maladaptive behavioral or psychologic changes that are due to substance effect on the central nervous system and develop during or shortly after use	2. Clinically significant distress or impairment in social, occupational, or other important area of functioning

252

2. Withdrawal Characteristic withdrawal syndrome for the substance or Same (or related substance) is taken to relieve or avoid withdrawal syndrome 3. Substance taken in larger amounts or over a longer period of time than intended 4. Persistent desire or unsuccessful attempts to cut down or control use 5. Inordinate amount of time spent to obtain or recover from effects 6. Important social, occupational, or recreational activities given up or reduced due to use 7. Use is continued despite harm	1. Recurrent use despite persistent or recurrent social or interpersonal problems caused by or exacerbated by effects of the substance 2. Recurrent substance-related legal problems 3. Recurrent use in physically hazardous situations 4. Recurrent use resulting in failure to fulfill major role obligations at work, school, or home	3. Symptoms are not due to general medical condition(s) and not accounted for by another mental disorder
	3. Symptoms are not due to general medical condition(s) and not accounted for by another mental disorder	

Reprinted with permission from the *Diagnostic and statistical manual of mental disorders*, 4th ed., pp. 181–185. Copyright 1994 American Psychiatric Association.

Individuals with SUD often are isolated, have poor self-esteem, lack impulse control, and possess a limited repertoire of healthy coping behaviors. The substance often becomes the primary relationship to the exclusion of other meaningful human relationships. During stressful periods (e.g., trauma, surgery, cancer diagnosis), an individual with SUD may seek support from substance(s).

Denial is a key feature of SUD. Minimizing use, downplaying the significance of the situation, blaming others, and diverting attention away from the problem protect the denial system. Individuals generally attribute their circumstances to something or someone outside of themselves and do not take responsibility for their own actions. Manipulation and hostility insulate the denial system, and an admission of responsibility would cause fragmentation. Attempts to control others trigger powerful emotions (anger, frustration, indifference) and serve to keep people at a distance. Interpersonal relationships suffer, and the individual is further isolated. Hostility is very effective in reinforcing the denial because people in a position to be helpful (i.e., family, friends, health care providers) will retreat.

Pain behaviors of an individual with SUD may be exaggerated. The exaggerated behavior is seen as atypical, excessive, and demanding and often calls into question the credibility of the pain report. The pain's intensity may be described in grandiose terms with accompanying physical gestures to reinforce its depth. Repeated and forceful requests for analgesic relief accompanied by attempts to make the pain as "real" as possible may have an unintended effect—less rather than more pain relief results.

SUBSTANCE USE DISORDER ASSESSMENT

A good SUD assessment should be part of all health assessments. The type and extent of information depend on the setting and patient's condition. The goal of screening is not to determine guilt or innocence. The objective, in the context of pain management, is to facilitate the establishment of a treatment plan that includes care to prevent and minimize withdrawal, address health concerns, relieve pain, and provide access to rehabilitative treatment.

Assessment data are collected through observation, interview (patient, family, review of medical record), physical examination, and laboratory testing. Patients may self-identify, demonstrate physical or behavioral manifestations of intoxication or withdrawal (Table 13–2), exhibit aberrant drug-related behaviors, and/or present with health problems associated with substance use (e.g., cirrhosis, pancreatitis, trauma, esophageal varices, myopathies, nasal septum damage, SUDs, viral hepatitis) (Lange, et al, 1992). It is important to remember that denial is a core component of SUD. Failure to recognize the problem and/or minimizing or downplaying the problem can be expected. Furthermore, denial can be sustained by health care professionals who are unwilling to address SUD.

Interviewing Strategies

The following provides some interviewing guidelines (Vourakis, 1994):

- Establish rapport.
- Question drug use in a matter-of-fact manner as one would ask about other aspects in a general health assessment.
- Begin with questions about over-the-counter medications, caffeine, cigarettes, prescription medications; proceed to screening questions for alcohol and illicit substances.
- If drug use is suspected, ask questions that presume and normalize quantities used. Ask "when was your last drink?," not "do you drink?" Ask "do you drink a 12 pack . . . a pint . . . a fifth a day?," not "how much do you drink?" Ask "when did you last use cocaine?," not "do you use cocaine?" Ask "what drugs do you mix?," not "do you ever mix drugs?"

Text continued on page 270

TABLE 13–2   Substance-Specific Intoxication or Withdrawal Manifestations

Substance	Signs and Symptoms of Intoxication	Signs and Symptoms of Withdrawal	Time Course of Withdrawal	Treatment of Withdrawal	Drug Screening and Medical Complications of Chronic Use
Alcohol	Slurred speech, incoordination, unsteady gait, nystagmus, attention or memory impairment, stupor, coma, bradycardia, decreased pulse, hypotension	Early signs: anxiety, restlessness, mild disorientation, sweating, tachycardia, hypertension, insomnia, nausea or vomiting. Progression to: hand tremor, transient visual, tactile, or auditory hallucinations or illusions, seizures (<3%) Delirium tremens (DTs): disorientation, hallucinations, tremors, agitation, increased autonomic nervous system activity tend to de-	Onset: 4–12 hrs few days after reduction of intake following heavy, prolonged use Peak: day 2 Improvement by day 4–5. Less intense symptoms of anxiety, insomnia and autonomic dysfunction may persist for up to 3–6 months Onset to DT often sudden; generally occurs day 3–4 after abstinence and lasts for 2–4 days	Pharmacologic management. Longer-acting benzodiazepines: chlordiazepoxide (Librium®); loading dose; then tapered doses over day 4–6 Clorazepate (Tranxene®) and clonazepam (Klonopin®) are also used Daily dose and rate/duration of downward titration depend on patient response and duration/dose of daily alcohol use Phenobarbital can be substituted for Librium®; is less sedating. Short-acting benzodiazepines may be more appropriate	Legal limit for intoxication 80–100 mg/100 ml. Laboratory evaluations: elevated alkaline phosphatase, gamma-glutamyl transpeptidase, mean corpuscular volume, and SGOT (AST) Chronic use: gastritis, stomach or duodenal ulcers, cirrhosis, pancreatitis, increased risk for cancer of esophagus, stomach, cardiomyopathy, hypertension, stroke,

256

velop with concurrent medical conditions (e.g., history of seizures, old age, liver failure, pneumonia, GI bleeding, head trauma, hypoglycemia, electrolyte imbalance, postoperative status)

in medically unstable. Shorter-acting benzodiazepines (lorazepam [Ativan®]) are used in the presence of liver disease. Anticonvulsants may be warranted. Nutritional support includes calories, folic acid, thiamine, B-complex vitamins and vitamin K if prothrombin time is decreased. Metabolic interventions to correct glucose, phosphate, magnesium, electrolytes and water. Use of withdrawal assessment scales are recommended (e.g., Modified Selective Severity Assessment [MSSA]) (Benzer, 1990, Lohr, 1995)

peripheral neuropathy, cognitive deficits, memory loss, bone marrow suppression

Table continued on following page

TABLE 13–2 *Substance-Specific Intoxication or Withdrawal Manifestations (Continued)*

SUBSTANCE	SIGNS AND SYMPTOMS OF INTOXICATION	SIGNS AND SYMPTOMS OF WITHDRAWAL	TIME COURSE OF WITHDRAWAL	TREATMENT OF WITHDRAWAL	DRUG SCREENING AND MEDICAL COMPLICATIONS OF CHRONIC USE
Opioids Morphine, codeine, coheroin, oxycodone (Roxicodone®), hydromorphone (Dilaudid®), methadone (Dolophine®), fentanyl (Duragesic®), meperidine (Demerol®), levorphanol (Levo-Dromoran®),	Maladaptive behavioral or psychologic changes: initial euphoria followed by apathy, dysphoria, psychomotor agitation or retardation, impaired judgment, impaired social or occupational functioning. Signs: pupillary constriction, drowsiness, coma, slurred speech, impaired attention or memory	Anxiety, restlessness, myalgias, nausea or vomiting, lacrimation or rhinorrhea, pupillary dilation, piloerection, sweating, diarrhea, abdominal cramping, yawning, fever, hypertension, tachycardia, insomnia	**Onset:** depends on half-life of drug. Short-acting = 6–24 hr; long-acting = 2–4 days **Peak:** short acting within day 1–3 **Subsides** over a period of day 5–7. Chronic symptoms of withdrawal include anxiety, dysphoria, insomnia	Withdraw opioids 25% decrease q 2 days (25% of the daily dose prevents withdrawal) Methadone (Dolophine®) has been used in the past) Catapres® (clonidine) is more widely used. Never use opioid antagonist naloxone (Narcan®) or mixed agonist-antagonist in agonist-dependent patients Withdrawal symptom management may require: Imodium® (loose stools); Bentyl® (abdominal	Urine screen positive for 12–36 hours after short-acting; several days for longer-acting Chronic use: glomerulonephritis, constipation, colicky pain, inflammation, and infection at injection site

propoxyphene (Darvon®), pentazocine (Talwin®), buprenorphine (Buprenex®)				cramps), NSAIDs (bone/joint pain), acetaminophen (headache), Librium® (anxiety), Benadryl® (sleep, antiemetic, nausea, vomiting)
Sedative-hypnotic, and anxiolytics Antianxiety: buspirone (BuSpar®), carbamates, meprobamate (Miltown®, Equanil®), benzodiazepines Barbiturates: secobarbital (Seconal®), phenobarbital (Luminal®),	Maladaptive behavioral or psychologic changes: inappropriate sexual or aggressive behavior, mood lability, impaired judgment, impaired social or occupational functioning Signs: slurred speech, drowsiness, incoordination, unsteady gait, nystagmus, impaired attention or memory, hyporeflexia, hypotension, bradycardia, brady-	Anxiety, tremor, insomnia, anorexia, nausea or vomiting, transient visual, tactile, auditory hallucinations or illusions, psychomotor agitation, fever, tachycardia, seizures	Onset and duration of withdrawal depends on half-life of drug, dose, and duration of use and presence of active metabolites **Short-acting** **Onset:** 6–8 hours **Peak:** day 2 **Resolves:** day 4–5 **Long-acting** **Onset:** day 5–7 **Peak:** week 2 **Resolves:** week 3–4	Chlordiazepoxide (Librium®) can be used. Start with a loading dose of about 25% of the typical daily intake and reduce over day 10–14. Very large daily benzodiazepine use (e.g., diazepam (Valium®) >400 mg/day) may require 30 days of gradual titration. Some recommend use of clonazepam (Klonopin®) for detoxification from alprazolam (Xanax®). Phenobarbital is drug of choice in patients with	Urine tests positive for short-acting 1–3 days; long-acting 7–9 days up to 3 weeks Chronic use: sleep disturbances, nystagmus, diplopia, strabismus, vertigo, ataxia, hyporeflexia

Table continued on following page

259

TABLE 13–2 *Substance-Specific Intoxication or Withdrawal Manifestations* (Continued)

SUBSTANCE	SIGNS AND SYMPTOMS OF INTOXICATION	SIGNS AND SYMPTOMS OF WITHDRAWAL	TIME COURSE OF WITHDRAWAL	TREATMENT OF WITHDRAWAL	DRUG SCREENING AND MEDICAL COMPLICATIONS OF CHRONIC USE
pentobarbital (Nembutal®), amobarbital (Amytal®) Barbiturate like hypnotics: methaqualone (Quaalude®), glutethimide (Doriden®), ethchlorvrynol (Placidyl®) Chloral Hydrate	pnea, pupillary constriction progressing to dilation if hypoxic, stupor, or coma			seizure history. Carbamazepine (Tegretol®) has been used	
Cannabinoids Marijuana, hashish, TCH (pot, grass, weed, reefer, hash, rope)	Intoxication develops within minutes when smoked; few hours when ingested	Irritable or anxious mood accompanied by tremor, perspiration, nausea, and sleep disturbance	Withdrawal symptoms have not been reliably shown to be clinically significant	Anxiolytic chlordiazepoxide (Librium®)	Urine tests may be positive 2–8 days (acute use) and 14–42 days (chronic use)

Effects last 3–4 hours. Because of lipid solubility effects may persist or re-emerge for 12–24 hours

Maladaptive behavioral or psychologic changes: euphoria with inappropriate laughter and grandi-osity, sedation, leth-argy, anxiety, sensa-tion of slowed time, impaired judgment, social withdrawal

Signs: impaired coordi-nation, conjunctival injection, increased appetite, dry mouth, tachycardia

Chronic use: bronchi-tis, shortness of breath, hypertension, immune suppression

Table continued on following page

261

TABLE 13-2 *Substance-Specific Intoxication or Withdrawal Manifestations (Continued)*

Substance	Signs and Symptoms of Intoxication	Signs and Symptoms of Withdrawal	Time Course of Withdrawal	Treatment of Withdrawal	Drug Screening and Medical Complications of Chronic Use
CNS stimulants Amphetamine (Benzedrine®, bennies, uppers), Dextroamphetamine (Dexedrine®, dexies, speed), Methamphetamine (Desoxyn®, crystal, ice), Methylphenidate (Ritalin®), Phenmetrazine (Preludin®)	**Onset:** signs of intoxication begin within seconds to less than one hour after use depending on drug and delivery method Maladaptive behavioral or psychologic changes: euphoria, affective blunting, hypervigilance, anxiety, tension, anger, impaired judgment, impaired social or occupational functioning Signs: tachycardia or bradycardia, pupillary dilation, hypo-,	Fatigue, vivid and unpleasant dreams, insomnia or hypersomnia, increased appetite, psychomotor retardation or agitation, intense drug craving, mood changes, including depression, suicidal ideation, irritability, emotional lability, impaired concentration Depression and suicide ideation are generally the most serious problems associated with withdrawal.	**Onset:** Within a few hours to several days	Chlordiazepoxide (Librium®) for agitation. Haloperidol (Haldol®) for paranoid thinking Bromocriptine (Parlodel®) for craving	Urine tests remain positive for 1–3 days Chronic use: depression, fatigue, weight loss, sleep disturbances, psychosis, paranoid ideas, drug-induced schizophrenia, hallucinations

262

Substance	Intoxication	Withdrawal	Onset of withdrawal	Treatment	Notes
Cocaine Coca leaves, coca paste, cocaine hydrochloride (snorted or injected), cocaine alkaloid (crack, coke, snow, flake, rock, superblow, topo)	**Onset:** signs of intoxication begin within seconds to less than 1 hour after use depending on delivery method. Maladaptive behavioral or psychologic changes: euphoria with enhanced vigor, gregariousness, hyperactivity, restlessness, hypervigilance, hypertension, perspiration or chills, nausea or vomiting, weight loss, psychomotor agitation or retardation, muscular weakness, respiratory depression, chest pain, arrhythmia, confusion, seizures, dyskinesias, dystonias or coma	Dysphoric mood, fatigue, vivid unpleasant dreams, insomnia or hypersomnia, increased appetite, psychomotor retardation or agitation. Depression and suicide ideation are generally the most serious problems associated with withdrawal. Can persist for months after discontinuation	**Onset:** withdrawal occurs within a few hours to several days	Chlordiazepoxide (Librium®) for agitation. Haloperidol (Haldol®) for paranoid thinking. Bromocriptine (Parlodel®) for craving	Cocaine eliminated within 5 hours, benzoylecgonine (cocaine metabolite) typically remains in urine 2–4 days after a single dose and 7–12 days with repeated dosing. Chronic use: nasal mucosal inflammation, necrosis, septum perforation,

Table continued on following page

263

TABLE 13–2 *Substance-Specific Intoxication or Withdrawal Manifestations* (Continued)

SUBSTANCE	SIGNS AND SYMPTOMS OF INTOXICATION	SIGNS AND SYMPTOMS OF WITHDRAWAL	TIME COURSE OF WITHDRAWAL	TREATMENT OF WITHDRAWAL	DRUG SCREENING AND MEDICAL COMPLICATIONS OF CHRONIC USE
	anxiety, tension or anger, impaired judgment, impaired social or occupational functioning. Chronic: affective blunting, fatigue, sadness and social isolation Signs: tachycardia or bradycardia, pupillary dilatation, elevated or lowered blood pressure, nausea or vomiting, weight loss, psychomotor agitation or retardation, perspiration, perspiration or chills, mus-	months after discontinuation			weight loss, seizures, perceptual changes, hallucinations, paranoia, cardiomyopathy, congestive heart failure, ischemia, arrhythmia, headache, vasculitis, pulmonary hemorrhage, infiltrates, renal failure, impotence, infertility

cular weakness, respiratory depression, chest pain or cardiac arrhythmia, confusion, seizures, dyskinesias, dystonias or coma				
Hallucinogens *Indoles* Lysergic acid diethylamide (LSD; morning glory, Acid, Cube D, sunshine, blue dots) Dimethyltryptamine (DMT), psilocybin and psilocin (mushrooms, magic mushroom) *Substituted*	Rate of onset, duration of action, and intensity varies *LSD:* onset 60 min. after oral use; peaks 2–4 hr; duration 6–8 hr *DMT:* onset 15–30 min. (injected, sniffed, smoked); duration 60–120 min. Begins with stimulant effects (restlessness, autonomic activation). Sequence of experiences follows: euphoria alternating	Not well described. A type of "hangover" the day after taking a drug has been described, manifested by insomnia, fatigue, drowsiness, sore jaw muscles, loss of balance and headache	Not well described	Maintain calm, safe environment Anxiolytics such as diazepam (Valium®) may be required Chlorpromazine (Thorazine®) for agitation and treatment of LSD-induced psychosis. Cautious use of neuroleptics, as neuroleptics lower the seizure threshold	Urine screen positive 7–14 days after use Chronic use: psychosis, depressive reactions, paranoid states, flashbacks. Risk of self-destructive behavior

Table continued on following page

TABLE 13-2 *Substance-Specific Intoxication or Withdrawal Manifestations* (Continued)

SUBSTANCE	SIGNS AND SYMPTOMS OF INTOXICATION	SIGNS AND SYMPTOMS OF WITHDRAWAL	TIME COURSE OF WITHDRAWAL	TREATMENT OF WITHDRAWAL	DRUG SCREENING AND MEDICAL COMPLICATIONS OF CHRONIC USE
phenethylamines: Mescaline (peyote) 3,4-Methylen-dioxy-amphet-amine (MDA; Ecstasy) 3,4-Methylene-dioxy-metham-phetamine (MDMA) Diiethyltrypta-mine (DET)	with depression or anxiety Maladaptive behavioral and psychologic. changes: visual illu-sions, enhanced sen-sory experiences, hallucinations, para-noid ideation, im-paired judgment, perceptual changes in a state of wake-fulness (depersonal-ization, derealiza-tion, illusion, synesthesias [i.e., blending of senses])				

Inhalants					
Aerosol propellants: fluorinated hydrocarbons, nitrous oxide (deodorants, hair spray, pesticides, cooking coating products) *Solvents:* gasoline, glue, paint thinner, spray paints, cleaners, typewriter correction fluid, acetone, lighter fluid	Signs: pupillary dilation, tachycardia, sweating, palpitations, blurred vision, tremors, incoordination Time course to intoxication is related to inhalant used; typically brief; lasting a few minutes to 1 hour **Onset:** rapid. Maladaptive behavioral or psychologic changes: belligerence, assaultiveness, apathy, impaired judgment, auditory-visual-tactile hallucinations, impaired social or occupational functioning Signs: dizziness, nystagmus, ataxia,	Not well described	Not well described	Neuroleptics and other forms of pharmacotherapy usually are not helpful. *Note:* Alcohol is a common secondary drug of abuse in inhalant use	Urine screen for hippuric acid (major metabolite of toluene found in airplane glue, rubber cement, paint remover and thinners) remains in urine 2–4 days. Chronic use: chronic encephalopathy, cerebellar ataxia, peripheral neuropathy, cranial neuropathy, visual loss, multifocal central and peripheral nervous system damage, nephrotoxicity, hepatotoxicity, pulmonary hypertension

Table continued on following page

TABLE 13-2 *Substance-Specific Intoxication or Withdrawal Manifestations (Continued)*

SUBSTANCE	SIGNS AND SYMPTOMS OF INTOXICATION	SIGNS AND SYMPTOMS OF WITHDRAWAL	TIME COURSE OF WITHDRAWAL	TREATMENT OF WITHDRAWAL	DRUG SCREENING AND MEDICAL COMPLICATIONS OF CHRONIC USE
	slurred speech, unsteady gait, lethargy, hyporeflexia, psychomotor retardation, tremor, muscle weakness, blurred vision, diplopia, stupor, coma, euphoria				
Phencyclidine PCP, Semylan, hog, Tranq, angel dust, PeaCe pill, and similar acting compounds, such as ketamine (Ketalar®, Ketaject®) and thiophene	**Onset:** Effects begin almost immediately after IV or smoking, **peak** within minutes. Oral peak occurs within 2 hours. **Duration:** of intoxication 8–20 hours; several days with severe intoxication	Not well described	Not well described	No known antidote. Treatment is symptom-driven. Seizure control with benzodiazepines. Sedate with benzodiazepine or haloperidol (Haldol®) for anxiety, pain, rage, aggression	Detectable levels 1 to 30 days after prolonged or high-dose use. Chronic use: depression, lethargy, lack of sexual drive, mood-sleep-appetite disturbance, anhedonia, amnesia

analog of phencyclidine (TCP)	Maladaptive behavioral or psychological changes: belligerence, impaired judgment, assaultiveness, impulsiveness, unpredictability, impaired social or occupational functioning Signs: nystagmus, hypertension, tachycardia, numbness, diminished pain response, ataxia, psychomotor agitation, dysarthria, muscle rigidity, seizures, coma

Adapted with permission from American Psychiatric Association. (1994). *Diagnostic and statistical manual of mental disorders* (4th ed.). Washington, DC: References: Gillman, A., Rall, T., Nies, A., & Taylor, P. (Eds.) (1996). *Goodman and Gilman's: The pharmacological basis of therapeutics.* New York: Pergamon Press. Lowinson, J., Ruiz, P., & Millman, R., (Eds.). (1990). *Substance abuse. A comprehensive textbook.* (2nd ed.). Baltimore: Williams & Wilkins. Miller, N. (Ed.). (1991). *Comprehensive handbook of drug and alcohol addiction.* New York: Marcel Dekker. Sullivan, E. (Ed.). (1995). *Nursing care of clients with substance abuse.* St. Louis, MO: Mosby.

Drug-Related Behaviors

There are multiple behavioral characteristics that should alert the clinician to the possibility of SUD. It should be remembered that the presence of a limited number of these behaviors does not provide a definitive diagnosis. A significant constellation of drug-related behaviors, however, is far more predictive of SUD (McCaffery & Vourakis, 1992; Payne, 1989; Portenoy, 1990, 1994):

- *Prescriptive abuse:* forging prescriptions, selling prescription drugs, obtaining prescription drugs from nonmedical sources, finding and accessing multiple prescribers with failure to inform provider about use of other prescription medicines

- *Multiple episodes of prescription "loss"* (e.g., "dropped in toilet," "washed in my jeans pocket"), inability to account for medications (e.g., "the pharmacy didn't give me all my medication"), multiple requests for early refills

- *Misuse of prescribed medications or therapies:* concurrent use of alcohol and/or illicit drugs, unsanctioned dose escalation despite instructions not to escalate, aggressive requests for additional medications, unapproved use of the drug to treat other symptoms, injecting oral medications, drug hoarding, tampering with infusion devices, multiple ER visits

- *Use of "opioid protection" strategies:* requesting specific brand name drug formulations and resisting generic formulations, history of therapeutic response to *only* opioids, reporting multiple drug "allergies" that severely limits choice of therapies, extreme resistance to multimodality pain therapies, waiting until end of appointment to make medication requests

- *Deteriorating functional and social skills:* decreased ability to function at work, in the family or socially; negative interactions with numerous physicians and health care providers

- *Frequent missed appointments or late arrivals to appointment*

Toxicology Screening

Toxicology screening raises multiple clinical and ethical issues. Confidentiality must be maintained. The reliability and validity of the screening must be placed in its proper perspective. It cannot stand as the sole determinant of SUD. While helpful in determining recent substance use as well as compliance with prescribed therapies, blood and urine alcohol and drug tests "are not diagnostic for alcohol or drug dependency nor . . . determine the possible severity or extent of that use" (Sullivan, 1995, p. 436). Positive screens do warrant a more intensive assessment. Until an in-depth assessment can be conducted, the identification of drug, daily dose, frequency, duration, drug combinations, and time of last dose should be assessed, if possible, as this information is critical in anticipating onset of substance-specific withdrawal (Vourakis & Bennett, 1990).

Detectability depends on the type of drug, size of the dose, especially the last dose, frequency of use, route of administration, individual variation in drug metabolism, body weight, hydration status, and sensitivity of the analytical method used. Urine contains approximately 100 to 1,000 times more drug than blood or serum. As an ultrafiltrate of plasma, urine is sufficiently accurate for drug use and metabolite determination and is the biofluid of choice for drug detection. Repetitive screens are recommended for clinical decision making (Lowinson, Ruiz, & Millman, 1992). Another issue related to screening is the fact that detectable levels of therapeutic doses of medications have not been well established.

Interpretation of results must take into account the half-life of the substance being tested (Table 13–3) and the sensitivity and specificity of testing methods (Sullivan, 1995). Toxicology screens (i.e., thin layer chromatography [TLC]) have poor sensitivity and specificity, but are fast and inexpensive. They are used

TABLE 13-3 *Half-Lives, Cut-Off Values, and Detectability of Drug Use*

DRUG	HALF-LIFE (HR)	EIA GC/MS CUT-OFF (NG/ML)		DETECTION AFTER LAST USE (DAYS)
Amphetamines	10–15	300	100	1–2
Barbiturates				
Short-acting	20–30	300	100	3–5
Long-acting	48–96	—	—	10–14
Benzodiazepines				
Diazepam	20–35	300	—	2–4
Nordiazepam	50–90	300	100	7–9
Cocaine (C)	0.8–1.5	—	—	0.2–0.5
Benzoylecgonine (BE)	6.0	300	50	2–4
Methaqualone	20–60	300	50	7–14
Opiates (codeine, morphine)	2–4	300	100	1–2
Phencyclidine (PCP)	7–16	75	10	2–8
Cannabinoids (THCA)	10–40	20–100	10	2–8 (acute)
				14–42 (chronic)

Reprinted with permission: Lowinson, J., Ruiz, P., & Millman, R. (Eds.) (1992) *Substance abuse. A comprehensive textbook* (2nd ed.) pp 431–432 Baltimore: Williams & Wilkins.

Note: EIA = Essay Immunoassay; GC/MS = Gas chromatography/Mass Spectrometry (Drug Screening Tests).

in emergency rooms to diagnose overdose. Chemical analysis by gas chromatography and mass spectrometry (GC/MS), immunoassay testing, and high-performance TLC provides excellent sensitivity and good specificity.

BARRIERS TO PAIN MANAGEMENT

KEY POINT

Substance abuse and dependency do not preclude the ability to perceive pain.

Individuals diagnosed with SUD experience pain and have the right to receive effective pain treatment. Undertreatment, however, is common among individuals with a dual diagnosis of pain and substance abuse because basic pain management assumptions are challenged and additional barriers created. Although the ethical obligation to manage pain and relieve suffering is at the core of a healthcare professional's commitment, biases and lack of skill related to SUD treatment are prevalent among clinicians. These and other such barriers affect the quality of pain management:

- Pain, as a subjective phenomenon, depends on believing the patient's complaint of pain, yet substance abusers are not perceived to be truth tellers.

- Physicians are reluctant to prescribe opioids or other controlled substances for individuals with SUD, because the burden is on the physician to establish that a medical problem exists that requires treatment with opioids.

- Health care professionals lack skill in identifying SUD, expecting a single indicator of SUD rather than a maladaptive pattern of substance use resulting in behavioral and psychologic manifestations and physiologic signs.

- Society addresses substance use disorders in three ways: (1) treatment of the problem with avoidance and denial; (2) belief that SUD is a moral defect requiring punitive action; or (3) perception that SUD is an illness. Health care professionals commonly view SUD as a moral issue.

- Individuals with SUD are viewed by health care professionals as "difficult, belligerent, and manipulative" (McCaffery & Vourakis, 1992, p. 17).

- Excessive pain expression often is presumed by health care professionals to reflect psychologic dependency, not actual pain.

- Health care professionals remain fatalistic about SUD treatment (Shine & Demas, 1984). They typically are in contact with individuals who have failed SUD treatment.

- Health care professionals equate providing pain medication to individuals with SUD with contributing to dependency, "feeding a habit" (Gonzales & Coyle, 1992, p. 248).

PAIN ASSESSMENT AND TREATMENT

Assessment

Pain assessment strategies have previously been described and do not differ in individuals diagnosed with SUD. A pain assessment includes a detailed history, physical examination, psychosocial assessment, and diagnostic workup to determine etiology.

KEY POINT

Practitioners must be careful to look for existing pathology even if they are convinced that the individual is drug seeking.

Treatment

When planning care for patients with SUD it is imperative to establish priorities. Initially, acute intoxication may need to be managed, followed by efforts to prevent/minimize withdrawal. Then, immediate health problems are addressed to include pain relief. Finally, problematic behavior is addressed and access offered to SUD treatment. Realistic goals must be established based on the recognition that the existence and severity of the pain cannot be proven, problematic behaviors may escalate if pain is not relieved, and SUD treatment is appropriate if perceived by the patient to be needed (McCaffery & Vourakis, 1992; Savage, 1993).

Understanding the etiology of the pain complaint is essential to determining appropriate analgesics or nonpharmacologic interventions (types of pain and specific therapies have been previously described). Care must be taken to use what is known about pain and pain treatment. There is a difference in the management of currently addicted individuals and individuals with a remote history who are actively engaged in recovery programs. Relationship to medications is qualitatively different between the two groups as well as compared to individuals without a SUD history (Wesson et al., 1993).

Analgesic Considerations

General principles of pain management apply to patients in pain with or without substance use disorder:

- Provide around-the-clock dosing for continuous pain to break the association between taking medications and obtaining pain relief. Breakthrough pain may be treated by PRN dosing. Frequent rescue dosing mandates a change in the scheduled dosage.

- Consider the use of patient-controlled analgesia (PCA) pumps in inpatient settings, either a combination of continuous infusion and on demand doses for continuous pain or on-demand doses for intermittent pain.

- Increase the patient's sense of control by informing him or her of dose, time interval, and medication used.

Opioids will need to be used in the SUD patient who experiences moderate to severe pain. Dispelling myths and explicating sound treatment strategies are of paramount importance. "Withholding opioid analgesics from chemically dependent patients with pain has never been shown to increase the likelihood of recovery from addiction" (McCaffery & Vourakis, 1992, p. 21). Portenoy & Payne (1992) concisely make their point: Opioids may be used effectively and safely in patients with substance use disorders when indicated for pain control.

- Utilize equianalgesic doses taking into account drug, route, and anticipated duration of analgesia.

- Titrate to analgesia or side effects. Stimmel (1989) advocates giving as much (parenteral) opioid analgesic as the patient requests as long as it is safe.

- Use agonist opioids (e.g., morphine, hydrocodone, oxycodone).

- Avoid use of opioid agonist-antagonist compounds (e.g., pentazocine, butorphanol, or nalbuphine) in known or suspected SUD. These medications will precipitate withdrawal in agonist-tolerant individuals.

- Never use antagonists (Narcan®) in an attempt to "prove" addiction or precipitate withdrawal.

- Avoid the use of "potentiators" which decrease itching and other side effects of opioids but have no effect on analgesia. Some believe that the use of promethazine (Phenergan®) will potentiate opioid analgesic effect and reduce the amount of opioid required. Promethazine has not been shown to increase the analgesic effect of opioids (American Pain Society, 1992).

- Avoid psychoactive medications that have no analgesic properties. Do not administer sedatives or anxiolytics as primary pain treatments in an effort to decrease or avoid opioid use. Sedatives and anxiolytics have little analgesic activity and contribute to the sedative side effects of opioids.

- Recognize that individuals who are tolerant to CNS depressants (e.g., opioids, alcohol, benzo-diazepines) will require larger doses of opioids and/or shortened intervals.

Nonpharmacologic Interventions

Use appropriate nonpharmacological interventions, such as invasive or noninvasive physical modalities and cognitive-behavioral therapies as described in Chapters 6 and 7.

Communication

Communication among health team members is essential to ensure that direction is maintained and responses from those who interact with the patient are consistent. It is absolutely critical to establish early on who is responsible for coordinating care. Although each team member will interact with the patient at various times, a single person coordinating all efforts is fundamental to ensure continued alignment with goals. The patient needs clear direction about who has the authority to prescribe and to determine the frequency of assessment as well as the treatment plan. Specify and limit who will negotiate; excessive negotiations should be avoided. "It is inappropriate for a patient to dictate an analgesic regimen just as it would be inappropriate for a patient to dictate an antibiotic or insulin regimen in the management of an infectious disease or diabetes mellitus" (Payne, 1989, p. 52). Plan regular meetings so that there is clear and frequent interdisciplinary communication, which is essential to the success of treatment. Any disagreement among staff about the management of the patient must be discussed openly in this forum rather than acted on or inadvertently communicated to the patient.

Setting limits and identifying boundaries are important parts of managing the patient with pain and SUD. **Be sure limits are in the best interest of the patient and not punitive; never use pain relief as a**

Text continued on page 282

I understand that my pain treatment will consist of the following:

• • • • •

1. I agree to take medications at the dose and frequency prescribed.
2. I understand that the nursing and medical staff taking care of me will ask me about my pain during my hospitalization. They will provide information to Dr. _____ and _____ . I will discuss changes in my pain treatment with Dr. _____ or _____ .
3. Dr. _____ or _____ will evaluate my pain, how well the pain medications are working, and whether I am experiencing any side effects at the following intervals: _____ .
4. I understand that Dr. _____ or _____ are the only health care providers who can prescribe or make changes in my pain medications while I am in the hospital.
5. I will consent to random urine drug screening.
6. I will consent to psychiatric and neuropsychologic testing as determined by _____ .

7. I understand that I am not to leave the nursing unit unless accompanied by a staff member.

8. I understand that the visitor policy is as follows:

• • •

9. I will protect the safety of my medications. I will not give my medications to any other person.

10. I understand that this document will be placed in my medical record.

11. I understand that failure to comply with the above may put at risk my continued pain treatment.

Patient: _____ Date: _____

Physician: _____ Date: _____

Renewal Date: _____

FIGURE 13–1 *Pain Treatment Contract. Source:* M.D. Anderson Cancer Center; Pain and Symptom Management Section. Houston, TX. Adapted with permission.

I understand that my pain treatment will consist of the following:

-
-
-
-
-

1. I agree to take medications at the dose and frequency prescribed. Any changes in the dose or frequency will be only at the direction of _____.

2. I will receive prescriptions at the following intervals _____.

3. I agree to come to all appointments as scheduled. I understand that my next appointment is scheduled for _____.

4. I understand that pain medication prescriptions will be supplied only at my clinic visit. I cannot request prescriptions by phone or writing.

5. I agree to receive pain prescriptions only from Dr. _____.

6. I will consent to random urine drug screening.

7. I will consent to psychiatric and neuropsychologic testing as determined by _____ .

8. I will protect the safety of my medications. I will not give my medications to any other person. I understand that lost or damaged medications will not be replaced. I agree to report stolen medications to the police at which time
Dr. _____ will make a decision regarding the replacement of stolen medications.

9. I understand that if I have any questions, unrelieved pain or side effects that I am to call ① _____ or ② _____

Phone number _____ between the hours of _____

_____ Phone number _____ between the hours of _____ .

10. I understand that a copy of this document will be sent to _____ (Primary Physician).

11. I understand that this document will be placed in my medical record.

12. I understand that failure to comply with the above may put at risk my continued pain treatment.

Patient: _____ Date: _____

Physician: _____ Date: _____

Renewal Date: _____

FIGURE 13–2 *Pain Treatment Contract. Source:* M.D. Anderson Cancer Center; Pain and Symptom Management Section. Houston, TX. Adapted with permission.

bargaining chip. Expectations and limits should be made clear, as well as consequences (Ellis, 1993). Use of a written contractual agreement can help to make the pain treatment plan explicit. Components of the written contractual agreement (Figure 13–1) might include:

- Goals of treatment
- Outline of treatment plan
- Expectations of patient and staff
- Consequences of not following treatment plan
- Staying on the inpatient unit
- Responsible staff
- Reevaluation intervals
- Consent to random urine drug screens
- Visitor limitations

Ambulatory Setting Considerations

When the patient is seen in an ambulatory setting, some additional considerations may contribute to effective pain management in the patient with SUD (Figure 13–2):

- Policy regarding the replacement of lost or stolen medications
- Policy regarding unsanctioned dose escalation
- Policy regarding early refill requests
- Expectations about follow-up appointments
- Indication of whom and when to call about medications, pain relief, and side effects
- Provision of limited quantity of prescription medications
- Provision of in-home medication supervision by professional home care staff
- Communication with all health providers regarding contractual agreement

CASE STUDY

Peter is a 44-year-old male diagnosed with hepatocellular carcinoma and cirrhosis with severe chronic visceral abdominal pain. He is referred to the pain clinic by his primary physician who is concerned about treating pain in SUD and requesting information about adjusting methadone maintenance dose for pain treatment. He has been in a methadone maintenance program for 3 years for the treatment of polysubstance abuse, including IV heroin. At referral, his current dose of methadone is 90 mg daily. He continues to use cannabinoids and nicotine daily. He has been incarcerated for alcohol-related crimes.

The treatment plan consisted of assessment by a psychiatrist and neuropsychologic testing; treatment for anxiety disorder with lorazepam (Ativan®) and depression with fluoxetine (Prozac®); ongoing communication with methadone prescriber (methadone was not used as an analgesic and dose remained stable); weekly outpatient appointments and limited-quantity prescriptions (appointments were gradually extended to every month); random urine screens; opioid titration from morphine 80 mg to 120 mg orally every 4 hours (he was prescribed the exact number of tablets required until his next appointment and instructed to bring any remaining drugs to the clinic); intermittent use of antiemetics and antiflatulents to treat concomitant symptoms; a celiac plexus block, which he refused (had had numerous liver biopsies and feared procedure); and written contract (Figure 13–1).

There were several occasions when his clinic appointments were scheduled for earlier dates than originally intended to accommodate staff schedule changes, and Peter brought unused medication as per the agreement. The contractual agreement was placed in the medical record and updated with each follow-up appointment. The emergency staff and outpatient pharmacy supervisory staff were notified of contractual agreement and responsible prescriber.

In the 12 months since referral to the pain clinic, Peter's care has been provided by two consistent health care practitioners. He has been forthcoming with information regarding use of cannabinoids (currently abstinent for 3 months with validation by urine screens). Urine tests have demonstrated presence of prescribed medications *only*. He has been responsible in keeping his outpatient appointments, has not requested early refills, never reported missing medications, has taken medications as prescribed without dose escalation, and has not engaged in any "aberrant" behavior, with the exception of continued cannabinoid use. It should be noted that much of his drug history and criminal history was not initially shared with health care providers, even with probing. It was only after he began to trust his two consistent primary care providers (physician and nurse) and recognized that his pain complaint was believed and that there was a commitment to treat his pain, that he was willing to share his polysubstance use history. He provided not only information about his own use but also information about the drug culture. The decision was made to continue his pain treatment outside of formal SUD treatment based on his continued psychiatric care and ability to comply with the treatment plan.

It is important to recognize that even with the best efforts of the entire pain management team, the patient may refuse treatment. Clinicians must not view these situations as failures, but rather as opportunities that were not embraced by individual choice. The learning is that substance abusers are really not unlike any other population of patients: there are those who participate and achieve clinical goals and those who do not. The focus must remain on effective pain management for everyone.

CASE STUDY

James is a 54-year-old male diagnosed with left forearm malignant mesenchymoma status post surgical resection. He has severe peripheral deafferentation pain in the left forearm and hand with motor weakness in the hand. The pharmacologic treatment plan consisted of 7.5 mg hydrocodone and acetaminophen

(Lortab®) prescribed quantity allowed for a maximum 10 tablets a day); amitriptyline (Elavil®) changed to nortriptyline (Pamelor®) then desipramine (Norpramin®); finally discontinued titration and tricyclic antidepressant trials due to reported urinary hesitance and retention. Other pharmacological strategies considered were carbamazapine (Tegretol®) (excluded because of limited bone marrow reserves), mexilitine (Mexitil®) (excluded because of a significant cardiac history), and NSAIDs (excluded because of gastritis history secondary to alcohol use). A written contract was used, and primary care providers, emergency room, and pharmacy were notified of the agreement. A physician and nurse were identified as primary care providers. A psychiatric consultation was ordered for evaluation of SUD and psychiatric diagnosis (consultation rescheduled three times, missed appointments three times). A TENS unit was tried, but James reported no relief. A diagnostic stellate ganglion block was refused. Over a 10-month period he missed four scheduled pain clinic appointments. He did live 400 miles from the clinic and had to rely on public transportation. Random urine screens were positive for illicit substances and prescription medications not provided by his primary pain treatment prescriber. A family friend reportedly "slipped" cocaine into his food or coffee, and positive screens for marijuana were due to "second-hand smoke." In addition, urine screens revealed medications not prescribed and were intermittently negative for prescribed medications. Prior to obtaining urine screens, he was questioned about the date and time of his last dose of prescribed medication. He admitted to "sometimes" taking more than 10 Lortab® a day and running out several days before his appointment. On several occasions James reported unusual circumstances regarding the loss or damage of medications. Because he often reported taking his last dose of Lortab® several days prior to his clinic appointment, interpreting his urine screens was difficult. Hydrocodone (Lortab®) would be expected to be present in his urine for only 2 days. Although the presence of a painful condition was never in doubt, these factors (urine drug screen, missing appointments, lost medications) called into question his ability to self-medicate as prescribed as well as his inability to safeguard his medications. A referral for SUD and psychopathology assessment was reinitiated, but James continued to be unable or unwilling to comply with scheduled appointments.

He was selective with the information he shared. It was only after a missed appointment that he told staff of a recent incarceration. He maintained that law officers "had it in" for him, that they had contaminated his urine screen with cocaine, and consequently, he was temporarily jailed for violation of his probation. With his permission, his probation officer was contacted.

Throughout, his reports of pain were believed. Multiple attempts were made to treat his pain without success. James resisted use of nonopioid and nonpharmacologic treatments. Pentazocine and naloxone (Talwin-NX®) were briefly prescribed, believing that there was less abuse and diversion potential. He became more aggressive in his requests for Lortab® and reported multiple side effects with Talwin-NX®.

Given his difficulty in complying with the treatment plan, pharmacologic strategies were no longer offered after 10 months of attempting to use them. After a discussion with his primary care provider, psychiatrist, probation officer, institutional risk management, and members of a multidisciplinary pain treatment team, a nonpharmacologic treatment plan was offered, including diagnostic stellate ganglion block, physical therapy modalities, psychiatric evaluation, and TENS. James refused the proposed treatment plan. He was dismissed from the pain clinic with specific recommendations about SUD treatment facilities within his community. Pain treatment recommendations also were provided to his local physician. He was given the opportunity to return for pain treatment in the event he changed his mind.

CONCLUSION

Clearly, providing pain treatment to individuals with known or suspected substance use disorders is a challenge, a challenge health care professionals will confront given the prevalence of pain and SUD. Attitudes and deficiencies in basic knowledge regarding pain assessment and treatment as well as lack of knowledge of substance use disorders contribute to the challenge. In addition to understanding generic pain management principles, it is necessary for health care professionals to be familiar with diagnostic criteria for SUD, substance use assessment and screening tools, signs and symptoms of substance-specific intoxication and withdrawal, time course and treatment strategies, and pain treatment strategies employed within the context of SUD. Above all, clinicians must set aside biases and uphold their ethical, professional commitment to manage pain and relieve suffering.

Clinical Accountabilities

1. Assessment for substance use should be part of all health assessments.
2. Base assessment on the fact that criteria for SUDs must be applied within the context of use.
3. Give acute illness precedence over SUD treatment.
4. Assure pain relief despite substance abuse.
   - Recognize that substance abuse and dependency do not preclude the ability to perceive pain.
   - Accept that SUD is a disease, not a moral problem.
   - Take care not to overlook pathology by being overly convinced that the individual's complaint is drug seeking.
5. Prevent or minimize withdrawal.
6. Recognize denial as a core feature of SUD. Manipulation and hostility drive people away and insulate the denial system.
7. When opioid therapy is the choice:
   - Use opioid agonists (morphine, hydrocodone, oxycodone). Avoid use of opioid agonist-antagonists (pentazocine, butorphanol, nalbuphine).

Clinical Accountabilities *(Continued)*

- Utilize equianalgesic doses taking into account drug, route, and anticipated duration of analgesia.
- Recognize that tolerance to CNS depressants (opioids, alcohol, benzodiazepines) will require larger dosages of opioid and/or shortened intervals.
- Differentiate between methadone maintenance dosing and analgesic therapies.

8. Establish realistic expectations and set/limit boundaries (never punitively).
   - Address problematic behaviors: neither tolerate the behavior nor reject the patient.
   - Develop a written contract with the patient.

9. Educate and include patient in control of pain.
10. Specify a single person to coordinate all efforts.
11. Ensure communication among health care team members and buy-in to treatment plan.
12. Identify resources.
    - Consult as indicated: pain specialist, addiction specialist, psychiatrist, physical medicine and rehabilitation specialist.
    - Provide access to SUD treatment.

BIBLIOGRAPHY

Acute Pain Management Guideline Panel. (1992). *Acute pain management: Operative or medical procedures and trauma.* AHPR Pub. #92-0032. Washington, DC: U.S. Department of Health and Human Service, Agency for Health Care Policy and Research.

American Pain Society. (1992). *Principles of analgesic use in the treatment of acute pain and chronic cancer pain* (3rd ed.). Skokie, IL: Author.

American Psychiatric Association. (1994). *Diagnostic and statistical manual of mental disorders* (4th ed.). Washington, DC: Author.

Babor, T., de la Fluente, J., Sanders, J., & Grant, M. (1989). *AUDIT: The Alcohol Use Disorders Identification Test: Guidelines for use in primary health care.* Geneva: World Health Organization.

Blendon, R., Aiken, L., Freeman, H., & Corey, C. (1989). Access to medical care for black and white Americans. A matter of continuing concern. *Journal of the American Medical Association, 261*(2), 278–281.

Burgess, M. (1980). *Nurses pain ratings of patient with acute and chronic low back pain.* Unpublished master's thesis, University of Alabama at Birmingham, Birmingham, AL.

Cancer Pain Management Guideline Panel. (1994). *Management of cancer pain.* AHCPR Pub. #94-0592. Rockville, MD: U.S. Department of Health and Human Services, Agency for Health Care Policy and Research, Public Health Service.

Clark, H., & Sees, K. (1993). Opioids, chronic pain and the law. *Journal of Pain and Symptom Management, 8*(5), 297–305.

Cleeland, C., Gonin, R., Hatfield, A., Edmonson, J., Blum, R., Stewart, J., & Pandya, K. (1994). Pain and its treatment in outpatients with metastatic cancer. *New England Journal of Medicine, 330*(9), 592–596.

Cohen, G., Griffin, P., & Wiltz, G. (1982). Stereotyping as a negative factor in substance abuse treatment. *International Journal of the Addiction, 17*(2), 371–376.

Cyr, M., & Wartman, S. (1988). The effectiveness of routine screening questions in the detection of alcoholism. *Journal of the American Medical Association, 259*(1), 51–54.

Daut, R., & Cleeland, C. (1982). The prevalence and severity of pain in cancer. *Cancer, 50*(9), 1913–1918.

Edwards, R. (1984). Pain management and the values of health care providers. In C. Hill & W. Fields (Eds.), *Advances in pain research and therapy* (Vol. 11, pp. 101–112). New York: Raven.

Ellis, N. (1993). Manipulation. In R. Rawlins & S. Williams (Eds.), *Mental health-psychiatric nursing: A holistic life-cycle approach* (pp. 235–257). St. Louis, MO: Mosby.

Ewing, J. (1984). Detecting alcoholism, the CAGE questionnaire. *Journal of the American Medical Association, 252*(14), 1905–1907.

Ferrell, B.A. (1990). Pain management in elderly people. *Journal of the American Geriatric Society, 38*(4), 409–414.

Fleming, M., & Barry, K. (1992). *Addictive disorders.* St. Louis, MO: Mosby.

Gonzales, G., & Coyle, N. (1992). Treatment of cancer pain in former opioid abusers: Fears of the patient and staff and their influence on care. *Journal of Pain and Symptom Management, 7*(4), 246–249.

Grossman, S., Scheidler, V., Sweden, K., Muncenski, J., & Piantadosi, S. (1991). Correlation of patients and care giver rating of cancer pain. *Journal of Pain and Symptom Management, 6*(2), 53–57.

Hedlund, J., & Viewig, B. (1984). The Michigan Alcoholism Screening Test: A comprehensive review. *Journal of Operational Psychiatry, 15,* 55–65.

Hill, C. (1993). The negative influence of licensing and disciplinary boards and drug enforcement agencies on pain treatment with opioid analgesics. *Journal of Pharmaceutical Care in Pain and Symptom Control, 1*(1), 43–62.

Joranson, D., & Gilson, A. (1994a). Controlled substances, medical practice, and the law. In H. Schwartz (Ed.), *Psychiatric practices under fire. The influence of government, the media, and special interests on somatic therapies,* (pp. 173–194). Washington, DC: American Psychiatric Press.

Joranson, D., Cleeland, C., Weissman, D., & Bilson, A. (1992). Opioids for chronic cancer and non-cancer pain: A survey of state medical board members. *Federation Bulletin: The Journal of Medical Licensure and Discipline, 79*(4), 15–49.

Knapp, D., & Koch, H. (1984). The management of new pain in office-based ambulatory care: National ambulatory medical care survey, 1980 and 1981. *National Health Care Statistics, 97,* 1–9.

Lange, W., White, N., & Robinson, N. (1992). Medical complications of substance abuse. *Post Graduate Medicine, 92*(3), 206–214.

Lowinson, J., Ruiz, P., & Millman, R. (Eds.). (1992). *Substance abuse. A comprehensive textbook* (2nd ed.). Baltimore: Williams & Wilkins.

Marks, R., & Sachar, E. (1973). Undertreatment of medical inpatients with narcotic analgesics. *Annuals of Internal Medicine, 78*(2), 173–181.

McCaffery, M., & Beebe, M. (1989). *Pain: Clinical manual for nursing practice.* St. Louis, MO: Mosby.

McCaffery, M., & Ferrell, B. (1991). Patient age. Does it affect your pain-control decisions? *Nursing 91, 21*(9), 44–48.

McCaffery, M., & Vourakis, C. (1992). Assessment and relief of pain in chemically dependent patients. *Orthopaedic Nursing, 11*(2), 13–26.

McCaffery, M., Ferrell, B., O'Neil-Page, E., & Lester, M. (1990). Nurses knowledge of opioid analgesic drugs and psychological dependency. *Cancer Nursing, 13*(1), 21–27.

McGuire, D. (1992). Comprehensive and multidimensional assessment and measurement of pain. *Journal of Pain and Symptom Management, 7*(5), 312–319.

Moore, R., Bone, L., Geller, G., Mamon, J., Stokes, E., & Levine, D. (1989). Prevalence, detection and treatment of alcoholism in hospitalized patients. *Journal of the American Medical Association, 41*(4), 403–407.

National Institute on Alcohol Abuse and Alcoholism. (1993). *Eighth special report to U.S. Congress: Alcohol and health.* DHHS Publication No. ADM 281-88-003. Alexandria, VA: Editorial Experts.

National Institute on Drug Abuse. (1991). *Drug abuse and drug abuse research.* The Third Triennial Report to Congress from the Secretary, Department of Health and Human Services. DHHS Publication No. ADM 9101704. Washington, DC: U.S. Government Printing Office.

Orsay, E., Doan-Wiggins, L., Lewis, R., Lucke, R., & RamaKrishnan, V. (1994). The impaired driver: Hospital and police detection alcohol and other drugs of abuse in motor vehicle crashes. *Annals of Emergency Medicine, 24*(1), 51–55.

Payne, R. (1989). Pain in the drug abuser, In K. Foley & R. Payne (Eds.), *Current therapy of pain* (pp. 46–54). Philadelphia: Decker.

Peebles, R., & Schneidman, D. (1991). *Socio-economic factbook for surgery, 1991–1992.* Chicago: American College of Surgeons.

Portenoy, R. (1990). Chronic opioid therapy in nonmalignant pain. *Journal of Pain and Symptom Management, 5*(1): S46–S62.

Portenoy, R. (1994). Opioid therapy for chronic nonmalignant pain: Current status. In H. Fields & J. Liebeskind (Eds.), *Progress in pain research and management* (Vol. 1, pp. 247–287). Seattle: IASP Press.

Portenoy, R., & Payne, R. (1992). Acute and chronic pain. In J. Lowinson, P. Ruiz, & R. Millman (Eds.), *Substance abuse. A comprehensive textbook* (2nd ed., pp. 691–721). Seattle: IASP Press.

Reyna, T., Hollis, H., & Hulsebus, R. (1985). Alcohol related trauma. *Annals of Surgery, 201*(1), 194–199.

Robins, L., & Regier, D. (1991). *Psychiatric disorders in America: The epidemiologic catchment area study.* New York: The Free Press.

Savage, S. (1993). Addiction in the treatment of pain: Significance, recognition, and management. *Journal of Pain and Symptom Management, 8*(5), 265–278.

Sees, K., & Clark, H. (1992). Opioid use in the treatment of chronic pain: Assessment of addiction. *Journal of Pain and Symptom Management, 7*(2), 257–264.

Selzer, M. (1971). The Michigan Alcohol Screening Test: The quest for a new diagnostic instrument. *American Journal of Psychiatry, 127*(12), 1653–1659.

Selzer, M., Vinokur, A., & van Rooijen, L. (1975). A self-administered short Michigan Alcoholism Screening Test (SMAST). *Journal of Studies on Alcohol, 36*(1), 117–126.

Shine, D., & Demas, P. (1984). Knowledge of medical students, residents, and attending physicians about opiate abuse. *Journal of Medical Education, 59*(6), 501–507.

Skinner, H. (1982). The drug abuse screening test. *Addictive Behaviors, 7*(4), 363–371.

Spross, J., McGuire, D., & Schmitt, R. (1991). Oncology nursing society position paper on cancer pain. Part 1: *Oncology Nursing Forum, 17*(4), 595–614. Part II: *Oncology Nursing Forum, 17*(5), 751–760. Part III: Oncology Nursing Forum, 17(6), 943–955.

Stimmel, B. (1985). Pain, analgesia, and addiction: An approach to the pharmacologic management of pain. *Clinical Journal of Pain, 1*(1), 14–22.

Stimmel, B. (1989). Adequate analgesia in narcotic dependency. In C.S. Hill & W.S. Fields (Eds.), *Advances in pain research and therapy* (Vol. 11, pp 131–138. New York: Raven.

Sullivan, E. (Ed.). (1995). *Nursing care of clients with substance abuse.* St. Louis, MO: Mosby.

Swenson, W., & Morse, R. (1975). The use of self-administered screening test (SAAST) in a medical center. *Mayo Clinic Proceedings, 50*(4), 204–208.

Taylor, A., Skelton, J., & Butcher, J. (1984). Duration of pain condition and physical pathology as determinants of nurses' assessments of patients in pain. *Nursing Research, 33*(1), 4–8.

Taylor, H. (1985). *The Nuprin pain report.* New York: Louis Harris and Associates.

Todd, K., Samaroo, N., & Hoffman, J. (1993). Ethnicity as a risk factor for inadequate emergency department analgesia. *Journal of the American Medical Association, 269*(12), 1537–1539.

Vourakis, C. (1994, May). *Cancer pain management in individuals diagnosed with substance use disorders.* Paper presented at the meeting of the Oncology Nursing Society, Cincinnati, OH.

Vourakis, C., & Bennett, G. (1990). Treating the drug abuser. In A. Burgess (Ed.), *Psychiatric nursing in the hospital and community* (5th ed., pp. 634–674). Englewood Cliffs, NJ: Prentice-Hall.

Weissman, D., & Haddox, J. (1986). Opioid pseudoaddiction: An iatrogenic syndrome. *Pain, 36*(3), 363–366.

Weissman, D., Joranson, D., & Hopwood, M. (1991). Wisconsin physicians' knowledge and attitudes about opioid analgesic regulations. *Wisconsin Medical Journal, 90*(12), 671–675.

Wesson,D., Ling, W., & Smith, D. (1993). Prescription of opioids for treatment of pain in patients with addictive disease. *Journal of Pain and Symptom Management, 8*(5), 289–296.

14
Collaborative Strategies

Teams, teamwork, collaborative effort—these are the words of the 1990s. And these terms are as applicable to health care as any other endeavor. Certainly, the very nature of patient care demands that various professions interface with the patient and with one another on behalf of the patient's care. The real question is not whether there is a "health care team" but, rather, to what extent the individuals who comprise the team actually perceive and carry out their roles as team players. Functioning in a solo role side by side does not constitute a team. Anyone who has ever watched a team sporting event knows that, although team members have individual roles, they act together for a very clear goal. It is that synergy that distinguishes true teamwork, the ability to value different skills, yet merge them to achieve a greater outcome. Nowhere is this concept more relevant than in pain management, where each separate profession/discipline is aligned with a common challenge that demands the best from each of them and from all of them collectively.

To build a case for the team factor, for collaboration between professions, one might ask the basic question: "Who is accountable for the relief of pain?" The patient who experiences pain and all that influences it positively or negatively? The physician who prescribes medications and therapy? The pharmacist who fills prescriptions and answers questions about them? The nurse who spends the most time with the patient and knows his or her responses to treatment? The social worker, the therapist, and so on? The answer of the future would be "the patient," giving the full ownership and control to the patient with support from the others. But, we are nowhere near this as a universal answer, so until we make more strides with pain management, the answer for now is "all of the above." It is of significance that "the team" in relation to pain management includes the patient, not only the health care professionals. Together they collaborate to solve the pain puzzle and establish effective coping mechanisms.

Collaboration may be defined in several ways:

- Working jointly with others, as with an agency or instrumentality with which one is not immediately connected
- Union or bond that produces synergism that results in a combined action or outcome that is greater in total effect than the sum of individual actions
- Joint communication and decision-making process among caregivers with the goal of meeting the patient's needs while respecting the unique abilities of all professions

It is noteworthy that energy is evident in each of the definitions, that each contains a message of cumulative effects that transcend single efforts. The potential for a positive working relationship and superior results is evident. However, it would be remiss to omit mentioning that often there are conflicts between the health care professionals themselves that arise out of different expectations and biases about roles. It is important for the health care team to recognize their own vulnerabilities, to set aside turf issues, and work toward a true team approach to quality care. For some, this is a given; for others it is a learning that will be rewarded when some initial successes are achieved. The following are some guidelines that may be helpful to such efforts.

BUILDING AND MAINTAINING
COLLABORATIVE RELATIONSHIPS

Team development is the first step and includes the following:

1. Identify members.

   a. Individual expertise.

   b. Common goals and interests.

2. Define the task.

3. Mutually establish responsibilities.

Appropriation of a "collaborative mantle" is the second step:

1. Begin with these underlying convictions:

   a. All team members have expertise.

   b. No team member has exclusive domain over specific areas of knowledge.

   c. Each caregiver has an ethical obligation to function as a moral advocate for the patient.

   d. Each caregiver is trying to provide excellence in patient care.

2. Establish credibility.

   a. Individual and collective accrual of knowledge.

   b. Observance of each other's clinical skills.

3. Communicate effectively.

   a. Physicians, nurses, and others can mutually define independent interventions, dependent actions, and interdependent interventions.

   b. Nurses can use their knowledge and expertise in a proactive way by providing accurate assessment of patient response to ordered interventions; clear request for treatment changes if pain management is inadequate; and clarification of orders if there is concern about the appropriateness of the intervention.

   c. Physicians can clearly delineate the rational for treatment decisions; the parameters for treatment changes

Construction of a collaborative history is the last step:

1. Become comfortable with changed role expectations.

2. Learn to be open to suggestions from other team members.

3. Develop confidence in the clinical abilities and decision-making capacity of other team members.

4. Consistently articulate issues and/or concerns.

The dynamics of the collaboration continuum change as members gain knowledge of and experience with each other.

EFFECTIVE COMMUNICATION STRATEGIES

KEY POINT

The nurse is usually in the best position to evaluate the patient's pain status and response to ordered interventions. When the patient is not receiving adequate relief, it is incumbent on the nurse to contact the physician for a change in those orders. The nurse should be prepared to advocate for the patient.

Pain Assessment

It is imperative for effective communication and intervention that pain be thoroughly assessed and communicated in an articulate and concise way. Information must include intensity and type of pain based on the patient's report using a visual analog scale, numerical rating scale, or other rating method commonly known to all members of the team. Location and duration or frequency of pain must be noted.

Response to Ordered Analgesics

Communications must clearly state the medication ordered, the dosage, route, and frequency followed by the duration and degree of relief obtained.

Dosage or Medication Changes

The individual communicating with the physician about potential medication or dosage changes needs to have knowledge about the following:

- Equianalgesia
- Conversion from parenteral to oral or oral to parenteral routes
- Efficacy of varied routes
- Scheduled versus PRN dosing
- Breakthrough pain
- Use of adjuvant analgesics

Reference and Research Articles

All members of the team should share new information so their collective knowledge is state-of-the-art regarding pain management.

Misconceptions

Addressing misconceptions is a salient point as collaboration is built on mutual understanding and respect.

One last point about collaboration, lest it be perceived as a fad or an option. Research on various patient situations has demonstrated that negative outcomes decrease as collaboration increases. It stands to reason that pain management can be significantly improved if all members of the health care team work in concert. As the team sets the standard for unbiased assessments, consistent expectations, effective communications, and more progressive techniques, pain management will enter a new era with improved outcomes.

So where does collaboration and teamwork begin? Who will step forward to champion the cause of pain management? The authors envision a historical day when hundreds of thousands of clinicians everywhere will step forward in unison, accepting the challenge. And the sound and symbol of that step will change the face of pain forever. Fantasy? No—if individual clinicians confront biases and collaborate to manage pain, the power of their collective action will accomplish what has been until now an elusive victory—effective, compassionate pain relief.

BIBLIOGRAPHY

Alpert, H.B., Goldman, L.D., Kilroy, C.M., & Pike, A.W. (1992). Toward an understanding of collaboration. *Nursing Clinics of North America, 27* (4), 47–59.

Bushnel, M.S., & Dean, J.M. (1993). Managing the intensive care unit: Physician-nurse collaboration. *Critical Care Medicine, 21* (9 Suppl.), S389–S390.

Glossary

Acute pain Short-term pain experience that demonstrates progressive resolution as the tissue heals; characterized by common physiologic responses (elevated heart rate, blood pressure, and respiratory rate; diaphoresis) and common behavioral responses (grimacing, crying, moaning, guarding).

Addiction (psychologic dependence) Pattern of active, compulsive drug seeking characterized by a continued craving for an opioid and the need to use the opioid for effects other than pain relief.

Atypical analgesic drug A drug that is not a primary analgesic but that research has shown to have independent or additive analgesic properties. It is used to enhance the analgesic efficacy of opioids, treat concurrent symptoms that exacerbate pain, and provide independent analgesia for certain types of pain. Also called *adjuvant analgesic.*

Analgesic Substance that diminishes the perception or experience of pain.

Biofeedback A process in which a person learns to control physiologic functions that are not ordinarily under voluntary control or that have become deregulated because of trauma or disease.

Breakthrough pain Intermittent exacerbations of pain that can occur spontaneously or in relation to specific activity in the presence of regularly scheduled doses of analgesics; also referred to as *incident pain.*

Chronic pain Pain that persists a month beyond the usual course of an acute disease or a reasonable time for an injury to heal or that is associated with a chronic pathologic process that causes continuous or intermittent pain for months or years.

Cognitive-behavioral technique A coping strategy in

which patients are taught to monitor and evaluate their own behavior and to modify their reactions to pain.

Distraction Cognitive strategy of focusing attention on stimuli other than pain or on the negative emotions that accompany pain.

Dose-limiting toxicity The presence of intolerable or unacceptable side effects secondary to analgesic therapy that limit the dosage that may be given.

Endorphin A group of endogenous opioid-like substances that are released at a signal from the cerebral cortex; attach to the opioid receptor sites and block the transmission of the pain signal.

Epidural Situated within the spinal canal, on or outside the dura mater (tough membrane surrounding the spinal cord).

Equianalgesic Having equal pain relieving effect; morphine sulfate (10 mg intramuscularly) is the standard of comparison.

First-pass effect Reduction in analgesic availability before the drug enters the systemic circulation due to the effect of hepatic metabolism on orally ingested opioid analgesics.

Imagery A cognitive-behavioral strategy that relies on mental images to induce relaxation.

Intractable pain Pain that is difficult to relieve or cure.

Intrathecal Situated within the subarachnoid space between the dura mater and the spinal cord.

Local nerve block Infiltration of a local anesthetic around a peripheral nerve for the purpose of generating anesthesia in the anatomic area supplied by the nerve.

Loading dose One-time analgesic dose given at the beginning of the pain experience adequate to reduce the pain to a tolerable level. Produces a serum drug concentration adequate for pain relief.

Neurolysis The injection of a chemical agent to cause destruction and consequent prolonged interruption of peripheral somatic or sympathetic nerves.

Neuropathic pain Process wherein pain stimuli are

transmitted from the periphery to the cerebral cortex via a damaged nervous system resulting in structural and chemical alterations that affect the nature of the impulses.

Nociception Process of pain transmission from the periphery to the cerebral cortex.

Nociceptive pain Process wherein pain stimuli are transmitted from the periphery to the cerebral cortex via a normal/intact nervous system.

Nonopioid analgesic Pharmacologic formulations that relieve pain at the peripheral level by interfering with the synthesis of prostaglandins; include aspirin, acetaminophen, and the nonsteroidal anti-inflammatory drugs (NSAIDs).

Opioid agonist drug Any morphinelike compound that affects the body by producing pain relief, sedation, constipation, and/or respiratory depression; stimulates activity at the opioid receptor site. Examples: morphine, hydromorphone, methadone, meperidine, fentanyl, codeine.

Opioid antagonist drug Compound that binds to specific receptor sites and blocks activity at that site; may displace agonist drug, thereby stopping its activity. Example: Narcan®.

Opioid mixed agonist-antagonist drug Compound that has an affinity for more than one type of opioid receptor and demonstrates agonist activity at one or more receptors and antagonist activity at one or more receptors; may precipitate withdrawal in a person who has been on pure agonist opioids for a week or more. Examples: Stadol®, Nubain®, and Talwin®.

Opioid-naive Limited exposure, if any, to the use of opioid analgesics.

Opioid receptor Opioid binding sites found throughout the primary afferents and the neuraxis.

Pain (1) An unpleasant sensory and emotional experience associated with actual and/or potential tissue damage and described in terms of such damage; or (2) whatever the experiencing person says it is whenever she or he says it does.

Pain behavior Anything a person says or does that infers the presence of pain.

Patient-controlled analgesia (PCA) Opioid analgesic delivery approach that employs an external infusion pump to deliver opioids on a "patient demand" or bolus basis; dosage is driven by the patient's need for analgesia and the pump's preprogrammed instructions to deliver on demand an identified dosage at specified intervals.

Physical dependence Involuntary behavior based on physiologic changes that is evidenced by withdrawal symptoms that occur if the opioid is abruptly stopped or an opioid antagonist is administered.

Physical modalities Therapeutic interventions that employ physical methods such as heat, cold, massage, or exercise to relieve pain.

Pseudoaddiction Iatrogenic syndrome of abnormal behavior developing as a direct consequence of inadequate pain management; characterized by behaviors that mimic dependency.

Psychogenic pain Pain with no known physiologic etiology or whose complaints are clinically judged to be in excess of the organic lesion.

Referred pain Pain experienced in a region remote from the site of the contributing organic component; common in neuropathic disorders.

Rescue dose Administration of an analgesic on an as-needed basis to treat pain that occurs in the presence of regularly scheduled analgesics; also referred to as *breakthrough dose.*

Substance abuse Recurrent use of chemical substances despite persistent or recurrent social or interpersonal problems caused by or exacerbated by effects of the substance; use may occur in physically hazardous situations and result in failure to fulfill major role obligations at work, school, and home.

Substance dependence Recurrent use of chemical substances resulting in physical dependence, tolerance, unsuccessful attempts to decrease or control usage, inordinate amount of time spent to obtain substance or recover from effects, and decreased activities of daily living because of use.

Substance use disorder (SUD) Pattern of behavior characterized by maladaptive patterns of substance use that result in clinically significant impairment or distress.

Suffering Unpleasant emotional response to the pain sensation.

Transcutaneous electrical nerve stimulation (TENS) A method of producing electroanalgesia through electrodes applied to the skin.

Tolerance Involuntary behavior based on physiologic changes that occur after repeated administration of an opioid; characterized by decreased analgesic effectiveness and the need for increased doses to provide adequate pain relief.

Index

Note: Page numbers in *italics* refer to illustrations; page numbers followed by t refer to tables.